The
Holistic
Beauty Book

The
Holistic
Beauty Book

Over 100 natural recipes for gorgeous healthy skin

Star Khechara

green books

First published in 2008 by

Green Books

Foxhole, Dartington
Totnes, Devon TQ9 6EB
www.greenbooks.co.uk

© Star Khechara 2008
All rights reserved

Design
Stephen Prior

Printed in the UK by Cambrian Printers.
The text paper is made from 100%
recycled post-consumer waste, and the
covers from 75% recycled material.

ISBN 978 1 900322 27 0

Contents

Dedication

For Mum, Ken, Dad, Nick (and Bex), Jodie and Kye (my family, you're all nuts but I love you).

For my gorgeous boyfriend Andrew Nash and awesome friends Charlotte, Seth, Trine, Eor, Midwinter, Julesy B, Peg, Joanne, Geka, Ashley and Alex Butler.

To all fellow potion-makers and in particular to those who are new to this exciting and beautifying craft.

For Veronika who is always cheering me on.

For Mother Earth.

"Beauty is not in the face; beauty is a light in the heart." – Khalil Gibran

Acknowledgements

Thanks to Steven Baker for my awesome author photograph.

A big sisterly thank you to my little brother Kye who is a great proofreader and grammar expert, and without whom this book would be full of my very unorthodox sentence structures.

Big thanks to Green Books, my publishers who took a chance on a whisk-wielding, geranium-scented potion-maker, especially to Amanda who has guided this novice author through the editing process (almost painlessly).

Also a huge thanks to all my friends who kept me fed and watered, and who gave me company while I was chained to my PC for many, many hours a day; in particular much gratitude to Joanne for the loan of said PC to which I have become very attached.

To everyone at *Funky Raw Magazine* and *The Mother Magazine*, thank you for asking me to write articles, without which I would never have taken this path into authorhood.

And to everyone else who has encouraged and/or congratulated me, thank you! You don't realise it but you have all kept me going when the task seemed too difficult.

A special thanks to Tom Rivett-Carnac who suggested I write this book in the first place, and dragged me along to Green Books one sunny day a couple of years ago.

Introduction

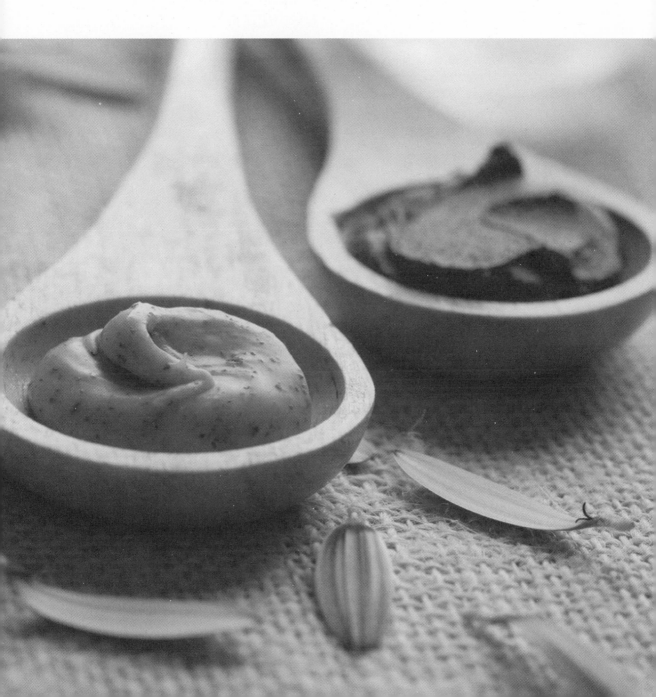

Introduction

SKINCARE WITH A 'CLEAN CONSCIENCE'

As a practitioner of holistic health and discerning earth-carer, I have great interest in environmental medicine: that which is concerned with the effect of toxins in the environment (air, food, water, cosmetics etc.) on human and planetary health. One of my specialist areas is the skin, and how to care for it holistically and avoid damaging chemicals; to this end I have been making my own 100% natural skincare products for over 14 years, and I now teach others how to make their own through my group workshops.

By making your own fabulous 100% natural Earth-friendly beauty potions you can lovingly care for yourself and this wonderful planet at the same time, although true holistic beauty comes from within and not from a bottle (regardless of what the label might say); being kind to your own body, the environment, plants and animals is an act of beauty in itself. Some say that beauty is only skin deep. Not so! Being a beautiful person inside is more attractive than having a 'fancy covering'; beauty is not just about what one looks like, but is a deeper expression of our personality. However, as skin is a vital part of the whole body, attention to its needs is also important.

To keep skin in a healthy state, and therefore looking good, depends on many factors including a natural water-rich wholesome diet, access to fresh air, and intelligent sun exposure. Using potions and lotions is only part of the equation; they cannot work miracles! In this book you will discover how to care for your skin in a holistic way and how to create your very own hand-made and totally gorgeous products that will feel wonderful on the skin, but won't harm planet Earth, its people or animals. Making your own skincare delights is also an enjoyable craft in itself, and is lots of messy fun for young and old alike.

NOT JUST YOUR AVERAGE BEAUTY BOOK

If you:
- are horrified at the synthetics, petro-pharmaceuticals, preservatives, toxic chemicals, colours, flavours, fragrances and slaughterhouse by-products that end up in commercial skincare products, even in those that are labelled 'natural'

- have sensitive skin or are concerned about using toxic toiletries on your children

- are unhappy with 'beauty industry' marketing methods, false claims and pseudo-science

- care for our amazing planet and the rights of the people, plants and animals that live here
- are concerned about the pollution of our air and water
- support fair-trade and are opposed to testing on animals
- encourage environmentally-responsible growing, harvesting and felling
- are interested in self-reliance and wish to live simply
- have a low-impact lifestyle and like to 'do-it-yourself'
- enjoy creating and learning green crafts
- love fragrant herbs, spices and flowers
- choose organic and local, but don't wish to pay a premium,

then this book is written for you. Enjoy!

HOW TO USE THIS BOOK

This book is composed of two main sections – one factual and one practical – plus a third section which is a resource guide.

For those who wish just to get stuck in and make wonderful lotions and potions that will make you glow, please feel free to whizz straight to the potion pages where you'll find recipes galore, plus exciting information about the natural ingredients to use and useful ideas and tips on how to package the finished potions in an Earth-friendly yet stylish way. Just as it isn't necessary to be a food scientist to know how to bake a cake, likewise it isn't necessary to study cosmetic science to make gorgeous beauty products that work. So if the 'sciencey bits' in the front of the book don't interest you, it is fine to skip them; you won't be 'cheating' and you will still have fun making great products that will delight body and soul! You can also come back to the theoretical bits another time once you've worn yourself out with all that whisking.

This book is packed with information about the hidden side of the cosmetic and beauty industry; there are chapters about skincare myths and toxic toiletries. You will also find a 'behind the scenes' look at some of the unsustainable and unethical practices of the herb and essential-oil industry to help you make ethical choices. Other environmental issues are raised here, with a look at packaging and how cosmetic ingredients affect our natural world. If you've ever wondered what the word 'natural' really means and what constitutes a natural ingredient or product, look no further. For those with an interest in whole body health, there are chapters that look at the holistic viewpoint of skin and its physiology, and at the link between nutrition, health and beauty.

At the back of the book there are the resources; here you will find useful websites, relevant campaigns and organisations, recommended reading and ethical suppliers of ingredients, so you can carry on up the potion path long after this book has disappeared under a mess of cocoa butter grease and oatmeal crumbs.

Be empowered and inspired, but most of all have fun, make a mess and feel beautiful without costing the Earth.

MEASUREMENTS IN THE RECIPES

UK readers

Use the first set of measurements (the metric ones).

North American readers

Use the second set of measurements (the imperial ones). The teaspoon and table-spoon quantities given after the slash sign (/) are the **US** versions.

In recipes where you want to use exact quantities in order to get the right texture, please note that where only **one** measure-ment in teaspoons or tablespoons is given, these are **UK** measurements, which are a bit larger than their US equivalents: 5 UK tea-spoons are equivalent to 6 US teaspoons (the same ratio applies to tablespoons). So you will need to add a little more.

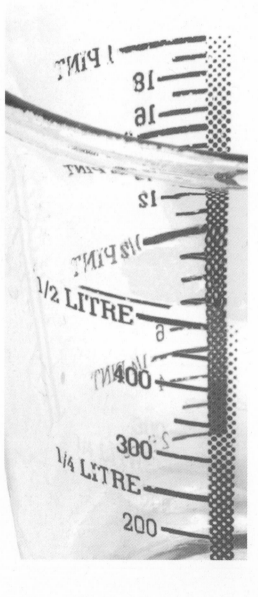

Chapter 1

Why DIY beautify?

Some of the benefits of making your own skincare products are:

1. You know exactly what you've put in it
2. You can tailor-make it for your own skin needs
3. You can make it smell the way you like
4. You can create a product with your exact ethical specifications (e.g. vegan, organic, fair-trade etc.)
5. Your potion is freshly made
6. You can avoid ingredients that you're allergic to
7. You can choose eco-friendly packaging and avoid plastic
8. You can make really gorgeous gifts that will impress your friends!

The main point to keep in mind, when making your own beauty products, is that the skin is part of the whole body and is actually our largest organ. You can only truly 'feed' the skin from within (by eating, drinking and breathing) and not through the use of external lotions. Treat your skin with the same respect as you'd treat your liver (also a large organ!). After all, if you wouldn't rub methyl paraben on your liver or eat it, perhaps it would be prudent not to apply it to the skin also.

JUNK (SKIN) FOOD

- **We know that processed, junk and ready-made packaged food is unhealthy, and that its convenience comes with a hefty health price.**
- **The same is true of your skincare products.**
- **Ready-made, processed potions are indeed convenient, but at what price for skin health? Junk products are always inferior to those freshly made from wholesome ingredients.**
- **Choose the home-made and the fresh over the preserved and processed.**

WHAT IS A 'COSMETIC'?

In legal terms, the word 'cosmetic' is used to describe a wide variety of personal care and beauty products. These can be roughly categorised into the following areas:

Cosmetics/make-up – Lipsticks, foundation, nail varnish, hair dye etc.: basically any product designed to superficially enhance beauty.

Personal care/toiletries – Functional bathroom products designed for daily use: things like soap, shower gel, toothpaste, mouthwash, deodorant etc.

Skincare/beauty products – Moisturisers, cleansers, bath treats, leg wax, face-masks, sugar-scrubs etc.

All of the above are subject to cosmetic law – in Europe, the **EU Cosmetic Directives**, which are long-winded pieces of legislation mainly aimed at makers of commercial cosmetics. However, just to give you an idea, the law states that the product must not cause harm when used for its stated purpose and that the responsibility for determining safety lies with the manufacturer. The Directives also list lots of ingredients that cannot legally be used or that have restricted use. However, as we will be using only safe natural ingredients we don't have to worry about that aspect, although it would be wise to familiarise yourself with the banned/restricted list if you are planning to make potions for others, as there are some natural ingredients on it.

Unfortunately the large cosmetic trade associations (which advise boards who form these laws) are themselves funded by memberships from large chemical and cosmetic companies, so despite there being a law about cosmetic safety, there are lots of very unsafe and downright harmful chemicals still legally allowed in skincare products. Even so-called 'natural' cosmetics often have their fair-share of nasties thrown into the mix.

The beauty industry itself is also very fond of using pseudo-scientific jargon to lead the consumer to believe that skin transformation of an almost miraculous nature will happen if you use their product. They also like to insinuate that their products are wonderful nature-potions mixed in the very Garden of Eden; this is because the word 'natural' sells, and it is very good marketing to get your customers to believe that a jar of petroleum, water and preservatives is actually a sublime blend of aromatic and healing plant extracts. Obviously, they can't actually lie in their adverts or on the label; however it is very easy to mislead; for example terms like:

'Younger-looking skin' – This is actually quite a vague term which can't be backed up scientifically as it is too subjective.

'Anti-ageing' – I have to laugh when I see this one. What are they actually saying here? Does a pot of mainly water and petrochemicals really have the power to halt time?

'**Hypo-allergenic'–** Most people believe that this means you can't be allergic to it, or that it is better or more natural and 'pure'. Not so! It literally means 'less allergy-causing'; basically the manufacturers have left out the most toxic allergens (allergy-causing substances) but have still made a chemical-based, unnatural product which could still cause an allergy or worse.

'**Dermatologically tested'–** How? And on whom? Under what circumstances? Does this make it a better or more natural product?

'**Pure'–** Another completely unproven, vague and meaningless term! Pure what, anyway? Would that be pure marketing? Or perhaps pure nonsense?

'**Aromatherapy'** – When the real therapy of Aromatherapy became popular, a lot of cosmetic companies jumped on the band-wagon and started making aroma-thera-peutic claims for their products. It is a very recognisable word, which conjures up images of fragrant plant extracts that beautify and soothe the troubled soul. Unfortunately it is just another misused word, and often these products do not even contain any aromatic plant extracts, botan-icals or essential oils whatsoever.

'**Natural'** – My favourite misused word! The cosmetic industry loves this one (along with Pure, Simple, Botanical, Organic, etc.). The word 'natural' actually has no legal definition within cosmetic law, so anyone can use it, and they do. My advice? Never, ever believe any product (commercial or hand-made) that claims it is natural without first checking the label. The label will tell the truth behind the marketing nonsense.

'**Extracts of . . . (insert fancy and exotic-sounding plant name)'** Manufacturers love to add a tiny atom of a plant extract to an otherwise hideous synthetic concoction just so they can state it on the label as an attractive selling point.

'**Derived from . . . (insert plant name)'** The worst offenders of this term are those makers of commercial natural products (the type you might see in health food shops) because it detracts the consumer from really knowing what they are using. For example: 'Sodium Lauryl Sulphate (SLS) derived from coconut'. So now the customer thinks that they are washing their hair with a nice extract of lovely nat-ural coconut. Unfortunately the truth is that SLS is one of the most common and poten-tially nasty detergents out there; it is used in shampoo and toothpaste and is known for its toxic effects (more about these later). As for the coconut connection, all SLS is derived from vegetable oil (usually coconut) anyway, but it undergoes lots of processing involving sulphuric acid before becoming a detergent and is therefore classed as a syn-thetic ingredient. Not sounding too fruity now, is it?

TOXIC TOILETRIES

After that little insight into the world of the beauty industry and its dubious marketing claims, let's take a closer look at some of the more common harmful ingredients found in skincare products, and find out what kinds of toxic effect have been recorded. When researching cosmetic chemicals/ingredients and the toxicological data for them, we can refer to what is known as a Material Safety Data Sheet (MSDS); this is the industry standard for providing information about a specific chemical or substance. These are easy to find online: either simply type in the ingredient name followed by MSDS (e.g. sodium lauryl sulphate MSDS) into a popular search engine such as Google, or look up the MSDS on a specialist website such as that listed in the *Resources* section of this book. The most important point to keep in mind is that an MSDS only gives information based on the industry use of that substance, so if toxicological data specifies that an ingredient is a known carcinogen or irritant, then this will be based on studies using the undiluted form of that product. It is imperative therefore not to take this data as relating exactly to a shampoo or other cosmetic containing a small percentage of the substance in question. An MSDS, however, can be useful for giving a picture of how toxic some of these common ingredients can be.

Just for interest, here are some extracts from the toxicological data from the MSDS of certain common cosmetic ingredients:

Sodium lauryl sulphate – a detergent found in most shampoos and toothpastes

- Skin contact could cause irritation
- Moderately toxic by ingestion
- May cause mutagenic effects

Parabens (methyl, propyl, butyl, and ethyl) – preservatives found in most skincare products

- Warning! Harmful if swallowed or inhaled.
- Causes irritation to skin, eyes and respiratory tract
- May cause allergic skin reaction
- Symptoms include: redness, itching, and pain

Propylene/butylene glycol – a petroleum-derived solvent which can penetrate the outer layers of skin

- May cause respiratory and throat irritation, central nervous system depression, blood and kidney disorders
- May cause nystagmus, lymphocytosis
- Skin irritation and dermatitis, conjunctivitis

- If ingested may cause: pulmonary oedema, brain damage, hypoglycaemia, intravascular haemolysis
- Death may occur

DEA (diethanolamine) – Acidity regulator used with other ingredients (e.g. DEA cocoamide)

- Product is severely irritating to body tissues and possibly corrosive to the eyes
- Amines react with nitrosating agents to form nitrosamines, which are carcinogenic
- DEA is currently under investigation as a carcinogen

Sounds scary, but please bear in mind, that it is not so much the individual chemical that will cause harm but rather that the daily systematic onslaught of several hundred of these ingredients over a long time will undermine the health of the body. Most synthetic cosmetic chemicals have only been tested individually and for short-term effects; no one really knows how these different ingredients and chemicals all react together on the skin and in the bloodstream day after day, for years and years.

It is also wise to consider that even some totally natural ingredients can cause harm too: stinging nettles hurt – and apparently hemlock killed Socrates! When learning to formulate your own 100% natural cosmetics, get to know your ingredients very well and when thinking of using a new substance or something from your garden always research it thoroughly – there are plenty of helpful websites, which are listed in the *Resources* section.

Chapter 2

What is 'natural'?

'Natural' is a difficult term to quantify, and everyone has their own idea of what constitutes a natural ingredient or product. According to the dictionary, natural means "existing in or produced by nature" and "not synthetic". Unfortunately there is no legal definition of this word as it pertains to cosmetics/toiletries, which is why we find that the most heinously chemical-filled cosmetics can carry the term, and why even the most self-proclaimed wholesome-seeming potion can also contain a whole host of unnatural irritants.

Using the dictionary definition, a natural ingredient would have to exist directly in the natural world, which would rule out all of the semi-synthetic ingredients that are 'derived from….' as these would not occur in nature. This definition would make all detergents non-natural for example. By the same definition, all natural products would have to be blended entirely from naturally occurring ingredients to be able to be labelled a 'natural' skincare potion.

Truly natural ingredients can fall into three categories of vegetable, animal and mineral.

1. Vegetable ingredients: plant-based items such as cocoa butter, almond oil, herbs, flowers, essential oils, nuts and seeds etc.

2. Animal ingredients: things like lanolin, beeswax, milk, honey and animal fats

3. Mineral ingredients: things like various clays and muds and possibly certain pigments.

A case in point: soap

Is soap natural, then? Well, admittedly there is a huge difference between commercially manufactured perfumed soap and that which is handcrafted using natural fats and essential oils. However, it would not be quite correct to label soap as 'natural', as it does not actually occur in nature by itself. Soap is the chemical compound resulting from a reaction between fatty acids and a powerful alkali (usually sodium hydroxide). Chemically speaking, soap is a salt. (A salt being the compound formed by an acid reacting with an alkali). This particular chemical reaction is called saponification.

For example:

sodium hydroxide + olive oil = sodium olivate

sodium hydroxide + palm kernel oil = sodium palm kernelate

As you can see, the resulting compound (the soap) is a totally synthetic man-made chemical; nowhere in nature does sodium hydroxide suddenly pounce onto some fat and turn it into soap! This isn't to say that we shouldn't use soap, just that the term 'natural soap' is very misleading as no soap is natural. Perhaps soap-crafters should really label their soap as being manufactured from only natural ingredients as opposed to the soap itself being a natural product.

There are also other issues to consider, as well as the naturalness of an ingredient or product, such as whether it has been organically grown or sustainably harvested, and other environmental considerations.

ORGANICALLY NATURAL

When an ingredient is labelled 'organic' it is meant that it is grown to organic standards of agriculture, and not (as in chemistry) that it is a carbon-based compound. But what is organic agriculture? Put very simply, it is a way of growing that avoids using chemicals, pesticides and artificial fertilisers on the soil or plants. In reality the definition is a lot more complex. When using organic ingredients it is important to make sure they are certified by one of the proper organisations that do this. Here in the UK the main organic certification body is the Soil Association; they have a very informative website which is well worth a look. They also certify products, including toiletries, and have quite strict standards; however, they do allow a certain amount of synthetics to be used in the formulation, and so Soil Association certification is not a foolproof standard for ensuring a product is totally natural.

It is well worth using organic ingredients, as not only do you avoid pesticides and chemicals, but also because more and more people are generally interested in buying organic products and it is an ever-growing market. It also makes for a more pure and holistic product if all the ingredients are not only 100% natural but also organically grown. Organic growing methods are generally a lot better for the environment too.

FAIR-TRADE

Unfortunately a lot of ingredients used in natural skincare are grown in faraway destinations, and with this in mind it would be ethical to try to source these substances as fairly as possible. Remember that fair-trade doesn't mean organic or even natural. However, in the Suppliers listing at the back of this book (p.169) you will find companies that supply ethically traded natural ingredients.

EARTH-FRIENDLY

I always try to ensure, as far as possible, that none of the ingredients I use have been linked to any ecological concerns; and that, once made into a product, it won't cause any environmental damage when it has been washed off the body down the sink and into the waterways.

Natural ingredients are often assumed to be eco-friendly by default; however, this can be far from the truth. Sandalwood oil is no longer considered ethical or environmentally sound as the tree is now on the threatened species list because of over-felling for cosmetic, aromatherapy and perfumery use. Once the oil is distilled, the wood chips are usually sent to factories where children make incense sticks. In the *Resources* section (p.169) there is plenty of information to help you make ethical choices about potential ingredients.

GROWING YOUR OWN

The most holistic way to source ingredients is of course to grow your own, which is perfectly possible with herbs and flowers, and even honey and beeswax! The next best thing is to source from local suppliers. Most regions have herb farms or small businesses growing organic products that could be used as cosmetic ingredients. Preparing your own home-grown herbs for cosmetic use is covered in Chapter 6, *Potion-making basics* (p.40).

WILD-CRAFTING

Gathering your own herbs and flowers from the wild is a satisfying task, but caution needs to be exercised. Over-harvesting has been known to cause certain plant species to become rare and need protection. It's a case of studying wild flowers and knowing which ones are protected by law, and it is also important to use intelligence and discrimination; nettles are obviously abundant everywhere and considered a nuisance plant, so gather to your heart's content. However, you may find yourself in trouble if you gather a clump of old-fashioned and hard to find sweet violets. It is also wise to gather plants only if you really know what you are doing; if you are unsure, please purchase your herbs from a supplier instead. Never risk your health or the ecosystem out of simple ignorance.

VEGANISM/VEGETARIANISM

All the potions in this book are totally vegetarian, and almost all of them are vegan and labelled as such. It is not at all hard to make vegan potions, as there are so many excellent plant ingredients with which to make skincare products – it's just a case of avoiding the few animal products that are used in skincare (honey, beeswax, lanolin, milk, animal fat etc.) For non-vegans, it's also very simple to make a wide variety of potions with beeswax, honey, oils and herbs. Even if you're not vegan or vegetarian, this is the best kind of skincare to make anyway, as applying lard, butter or other animal extracts to the skin is not particularly beneficial or pleasant!

Chapter 3

Essential oils

Essential oils are ubiquitous in the world of skincare and yet remain a mystery to many, which is why I have dedicated an entire chapter to them. So what exactly are essential oils, anyway? Basically speaking they are volatile aromatic compounds which have been extracted from plants using steam or water distillation. Oils extracted using solvents (e.g. Jasmine Absolute) or by mechanical pressure (e.g. Orange-peel oil) may also be classed as essential oils. Flowers, leaves, wood and tree resins can all yield essential oils, and the viscosity, colour and price of the different oils can vary immensely. Some plants (e.g. Rose or Melissa) yield very little essential oil, and it can take several tons of plant material to make a few kilos of oil; as a result these oils have a high price. If the oil is available cheaply, then it is best to assume that it is not the real thing.

Most of us probably associate the use of essential oils with aromatherapy. However, the essential oils market is actually controlled by the perfume, pharmaceutical and food industries. Does this matter? Yes: because these particular industries are not interested in 100% purity, they need oils to be the same year after year, which is impossible when dealing with a natural product. You cannot 'standardise' nature. So the oils are adulterated, blended, de-terpenated, fractionated and generally altered to create the perfect oil for their needs. Because these industries control almost the whole market, it means that a very high proportion of essential oils on sale, whether or not they are labelled '100% pure', are not totally genuine. Most aromatherapy oil suppliers simply buy the oils wholesale from a big distributor so it is nigh on impossible to ensure purity.

It's not just the big businesses messing with these precious gifts of nature; the process of distillation itself can change the chemical structures within the oils and create new compounds. Exposing living matter to intense heat can change natural and benign nutrients into new substances which may turn out to be toxic to the body. Distillation is no different: when the plants are 'cooked', new chemicals can be formed that were not present in the plant before. Personally I love essential oils, and I'm certainly not saying we shouldn't use them; I just think it's important to remember that we are dealing with very potent, concentrated, heated, probably adulterated, extracted chemical compounds which may contain all sorts of new substances or impurities as a result of processing. Use sparingly, use wisely, and if you cannot be sure that you are using 100% pure oils then it's probably best not to use them at all.

If you are pregnant or breastfeeding, you need to be careful which essential oils to use – see Chapter 6, *Potion-making basics* (p.40).

INFUSED OILS

An alternative to using bought essential oils is to make your own infused oils instead; these are more akin to a ready diluted essence rather that a powerful concentrate. A good reason for making your own infused essences is an environmental one; I have always found it strange that whole fields of flowers can be destroyed to make a small amount of concentrated product that we then have to dilute! The wastefulness makes me cringe. The ecological downsides of essential oils can be shocking, and that's before we even consider the unethical and unsustainable felling of beautiful old sandalwood and rosewood trees. A lot of oils come from poor and third-world countries: is our desire for fragrance ensuring that others live in stink and misery? It is not as if our lives depend on using these potent essences – we can enjoy the simple pleasures of aromatherapy by breathing in the aromas of actual flowers and herbs. Take time out to smell the roses, feel the silky cool petals against your face and breathe in deeply; this is real-life aromatherapy!

An infused oil is a plant oil that has been infused with an aromatic or medicinal plant. The plant material is placed into a glass or ceramic container and covered with the oil and left to 'infuse' or 'macerate' until the oil takes up the fragrance and colour of the original plant; this usually takes about two weeks. The result is an already dilute oil which can be used exactly as it is for massage, in the bath or as a skincare oil, and it can also be used as an ingredient in cosmetic preparations such as creams and moisturisers. Depending on how much you want to make, all you need is a handful or two of fresh (dried will suffice) herbs or flowers and enough plant oil to cover them. It is easy, fun, cheap and anyone can make wonderful fragranced oils this way. You also have peace of mind in knowing that it is 100% pure and totally natural; and you can even use your own plants if you have some growing in the garden.

HOW TO MAKE YOUR SCENTED OILS

The general idea is to stuff as much fresh or dried plant material into the jar as you can fit, then cover it with a mild-smelling plant oil – sunflower, almond and apricot are all good – put a lid on the jar, and leave in a warm place (sunny windowsill, airing cupboard, radiator top etc). Shake the jar every day, and check weekly to see if the oil is nicely scented and coloured; this usually takes at least two weeks. Also check for rotten plant bits – some plants go brown and bits may need to be removed and replaced with new. If you are using fresh flowers or herbs rather than dried, then you will need to change the plants every few days to ensure you don't make mould-infused oil!

When the oil is suitably infused, strain it off through a muslin-lined sieve, making sure that any sediment in the jar gets left behind. Put your beautiful aromatic oil into an amber glass bottle and store in a dry, cool place out of direct light. It should keep from six months to a year.

Let's run through the process by making infused rose oil:

Infused rose oil

Ingredients
- Several handfuls of fresh scented dried rose petals
- 500ml/1 pint organic almond or sunflower oil

Shelf-life
- Infused oils keep for 6-12 months

Skin types
- Suitable for all, but especially beneficial for dry and mature skins

How to make
- Pack your rose petals into a large clean dry glass jar completely cover with the almond oil
- Put the lid on and shake
- Leave somewhere warm to infuse
- Shake the oil every day and check for rotten petals
- If any petals go brown, remove and replace with fresh ones
- Repeat until oil smells lovely and rosy (no longer than a month)
- Strain off your gorgeous rose oil through a muslin-lined sieve
- Put into a clean dry glass bottle.
- Label and date it

Use this luxurious oil on face and body, in the bath or in your home-made potions; feel like a gorgeous rose fairy with the softest skin ever!

This format can be applied to making any infused oil from a wide variety of medicinal and scented plants. Commonly used macerated/infused oils in natural cosmetics are:

- **Calendula oil** – fresh or dried pot marigold petals infused in oil
- **Carrot oil** – freshly grated carrot infused in sunflower oil for a beta-carotene-rich ingredient
- **Yarrow oil** – a garden lawn 'weed', yarrow makes a super skin-healing-oil

For those of you who would like to replace essential oils with infused versions, it is also possible to make up nice mixtures to replicate a diluted essential-oil blend, e.g.

- Cinnamon sticks and freshly grated orange peel in almond oil

- Rose geranium leaves, jasmine flowers and gardenia blossoms all from the garden!

- Fresh lavender buds, chamomile flowers and honeysuckle flowers

The only limit is your imagination, and what you can grow or buy.

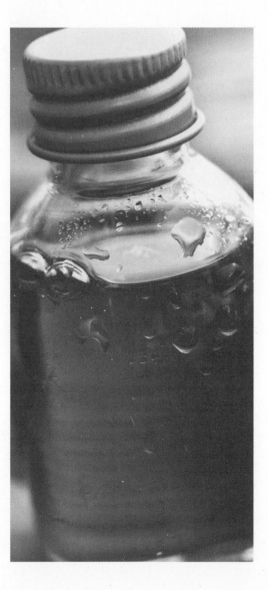

Chapter 4

Your intelligent skin

What sort of beauty book would this be if we didn't learn a little bit about the amazing body part we call 'skin'?

The skin is actually our biggest organ, and performs many important functions. It helps to regulate body temperature; the bacterial colonies on its surface form part of our immune system; it is one of our important organs of elimination – sweating out toxins and waste products from the body; and it is an environmental barrier preventing our water-rich bodies from drying out. Sensory nerves are abundant in the skin, making it an invaluable organ of touch. Our skin, when stimulated by ultra-violet light, also produces the pigment melanin – this darkens the skin to protect it from sun-damage. The skin also has a limited capacity to absorb substances applied topically, and amazingly even produces its own moisturiser called sebum.

The skin is roughly divided into two layers, like an open sandwich of very thick bread and a thin topping. The bread is the dermis and the thin topping is the epidermis.

The dermis is the main body of the skin, and is a tough elastic layer housing important structures of blood vessels, lymph vessels, sensory nerve endings, sweat glands and ducts, hairs and their muscles and sebaceous glands which produce sebum.

The epidermis is the bit we see and the part we cover in various skincare preparations, so we need to understand accurately what is happening in it. The epidermis is constructed of four layers, which are:

- The horny layer *(stratum corneum)*
- The granular layer *(stratum granulosum)*
- The prickle-cell layer *(stratum spinosum)*
- The basal cell layer *(stratum germinativum)*

These four layers are basically describing the journey a skin cell takes, from being all new, plump and shiny at the bottom to becoming a flattened, hardened disc at the top that is ready to be sloughed off. These flat dry outer skin cells, known as squames, are what we see and collectively refer to as our 'skin'; they are composed almost entirely of a hard protein called keratin. The reason that our outer skin is constructed from these hard dry cells is for our protection. Our living cells are about 80% water, whereas normal air is only about 1% water; should a living cell make direct contact with air, it would shrivel up and die. So our body intelligently surrounds itself with a layer of dry dead cells to protect the water-rich living ones. This horny layer is continuously being shed (desquamation) and new cells are always forming in the basal layer. It takes around 40 days for the epidermis to be completely replaced. This is important to bear in mind when working to improve the look of your skin.

Both skin and hair are normally kept healthy, shiny and supple by sebum, a natural emollient secreted by the sebaceous glands. This substance is composed of fatty acids, fatty alcohols and esters (waxes) which make a kind of light grease which waterproofs the skin, helps to retain moisture within the skin and imparts a healthy sheen to skin and hair. Sebum also contains natural salts and lactic acid which help to maintain the natural and slightly acidic pH (4.5 to 6) of skin and hair. Where there is over- or under-production of sebum, this will result in either greasy or dry skin/hair.

SKIN TYPES

Most of us are familiar with the concept and usual descriptions of 'skin types'. We either have dry, oily, combination or normal skin – right? Unfortunately, skin isn't that easy to fit in a labelled box! Most of us will have different types of skin on different areas of our bodies anyway, and for good reason. Considering that skin is constantly renew-ing itself every 40 days, our skin type could change several times. There may be environmental reasons for being a certain 'skin type': for example, the harsh detergents in washing-up liquid could be causing dry skin on the hands, which could be easily remedied.

Skin types are not static, but rather a snapshot of what state the skin is in at that present moment. The natural state for everybody's skin is for it to be healthy – not dry, not oily, not breaking out in pustules. If these symptoms exist, it is not because that is your 'type' but rather that your skin needs some help as it is not being given what it needs to maintain its state of health.

When creating and using 100% natural pure products it is not even really necessary to be concerned with skin types, as most ingredients will be suitable for all skins. However, for interest, here's a description of the traditional skin types:

Dry – has visible dry flakes, the skin may feel rough to the touch and itchy, feels tight after washing. May also be sensitive.

Oily/greasy – very shiny skin prone to break-outs of spots and blackheads.

Combination – oily 'T'zone (forehead, nose and chin), dry or normal elsewhere.

Normal – babies and children have this, most adults have to aim for it and take certain steps to achieve it!

We could also add a fifth type, that of sensitive skin. This skin is prone to allergic breakouts and rashes and can be very reactive to new skincare products, even those which are 100% natural.

CARING FOR SKIN HOLISTICALLY

It is important to understand that the skin, like every other part of the body, is self-repairing, self-maintaining and exclusively constructed using materials from our daily diet. Our skincare products can only do so much, no matter how natural and organic they are. We are literally built from the raw materials we consume, so if we want super-healthy flawless skin, we have to eat a super-healthy flawless diet high in water-rich, nutrient-rich fresh natural foods. Our skincare products are only playing a secondary part in creating the health and good looks of our skin. The best thing we can do for our skin is feed it healthily from the inside, and cleanse and nourish it from the outside with a few carefully formulated 100% natural safe products.

When deciding what products to make or use, it is a good idea to bear in mind these two concepts:

1. Less is more; the fewer products and the fewer ingredients in each product, the better for your skin

2. If you wouldn't be able to eat it, don't put it on your skin

This last one seems obvious, and yet how many people each day rub several toxic chemicals onto their skin? Nobody would dream of eating make-up, and yet it often gets worn on the face for eight hours or more. Remember, the skin is not a separate entity but an important part of the whole body and our biggest organ. So if you wouldn't rub shampoo onto your liver, it's probably best not to wash your hair with it. Although the skin only has a limited absorptive capacity, it is unknown exactly what that capacity actually is for each individual chemical.

LESS IS MORE

Considering that the skin has its own physiological processes that help to keep it in good working order, it is safe to assume that it needs very little in the way of lotions and potions to maintain its health. It is therefore truly astounding how many different skincare products are available; there are even different products for each individual area and part of the body. To put it simply, all we really need is something to clean the skin and perhaps something to moisturise it afterwards.

However, most of us enjoy using luxury skin treats and bath potions, and there are also personal care items to consider, such as toothpaste and deodorant, which have become necessary items of daily use for most people. On the whole it is possible to make fairly generic products (a hand cream becomes a foot balm which is also a rough skin-soother for elbows etc.) to cover a wide range of uses, thus cutting down on the amount of different ingredients that skin is exposed to. Why is this important? Well, just as in the diet, where the body assimilates most easily those meals made of fewer ingredients, the skin may also absorb and utilise those potions better which are made of fewer and simpler natural ingredients. The less the body is exposed to at one time, the less likely there will be an allergic reaction. It will also be easier to pinpoint any sensitivity to ingredients the fewer there are.

SKIN ENEMIES

We've all been subject to endless warnings about sun exposure, skin cancer and sun ageing. Yet the other equally important factors involved have been totally ignored. There are many enemies of the skin in modern life, and although we cannot totally avoid them all, we can protect ourselves from some of them and take certain preventative measures.

We cannot do much about air pollution if we live in a city, but we can choose to eat a better diet and thus make our skin more resilient to toxins.

Diet

This is by far the most important factor in skin health: please remember that every cell (including skin cells) in the body is built from the food we eat. A diet of quality natural foods will create healthy skin, whereas a diet of processed junk, too much salt, sugar, alcohol and smoking will create puffy, saggy dull skin prone to irritation.

Just making one dietary change – to drink two litres (two U.S. quarts) of water a day – will improve the skin immeasurably. There is more in-depth information in Chapter 5 (p.29), which covers nutritional advice for beautiful healthy skin.

Chemical exposure

Do you wear rubber gloves when you wash up? If not, your hands are being daily exposed to very drying detergents. Most people's hands are exposed to a staggering array of different skin-damaging chemicals in an average day, including the ones in their petro-chemical moisturiser they slather on afterwards to 'help'. It is really no wonder that the hands are usually the first body part to give a person's real age away.

Air pollution

Unfortunately, apart from campaigning about it, there's little we can do about the toxic air we all have to breathe in. However, we can help our skin by washing all the outdoor smog off when we come in. We can also make sure we are not adding to the problem by using chemicals in the home and thus polluting our indoor air too. Swap chemical room perfumers for essential oils instead, and always let fresh air circulate in the home.

Smoking

Nothing ages facial skin like smoking. To avoid greying sallow skin and wrinkles around the mouth, try to give it up.

Lack of sleep

It's not called 'beauty sleep' for nothing! It is really important that the body and mind get plenty of rest and quality sleep. The amount needed depends on the individual; personally I'm a ten-hours-a-night girl – any less and I instantly look older.

Clothing

OK, I'm not going to advocate naturism here, but seriously: how much naked exposure does your skin actually get on a daily basis? Skin needs to breathe, and being bundled up all the time inhibits the skin's natural respiration. The worst clothing by far is that made from synthetic fibres (nylon, polyester etc.)

Organic plant fibres such as cotton and hemp are the best, next to nakedness of course. Try to allow some time each day where you can be free of most, if not all, of your clothing. Sleeping naked is very beneficial, as this is when the skin is busy repairing itself.

Indoor life

Our skin is designed to be exposed to the elements, but sadly most of us spend a lot of our time not only covered up in artificial fabric but also ensconced cosily inside stuffy overheated rooms. Central heating and air-conditioning all have a drying effect on the skin, making it more prone to ill-health and forming wrinkles. Turning down the heating and opening some windows to let fresh air in will brighten up the complexion and is a positive step towards healthy skin.

Make-up

Often, skin issues can be traced back to over-use of make-up. It is simply just not natural for the skin to be coated in a thick layer of pigments every single day; not only does this clog up the tiny pores and prevent the skin from breathing properly, but there is the added downside of negative effects from the chemicals in those cosmetics. For beautiful healthy skin, go to bed without wearing make-up or skincare products. If, during the daytime, make-up really must be worn, then look out for one of those new companies which make cosmetics using earth pigments and natural waxes instead of synthetic substances and animal fats.

This is quite a list, but don't panic and try to change everything at once. Just be mindful of the potential skin enemies linked to your own lifestyle and gradually adjust accordingly. It's the tweaking of these seemingly small matters that can make a big difference to your skin. Maybe pick one 'skin enemy' a month to tackle: e.g. start wearing rubber gloves whenever you wash up or clean the house. Once this habit is formed, move on to sorting out your sleeping habits etc. It won't take long to turn your lifestyle into one that supports whole body health and skin beautification.

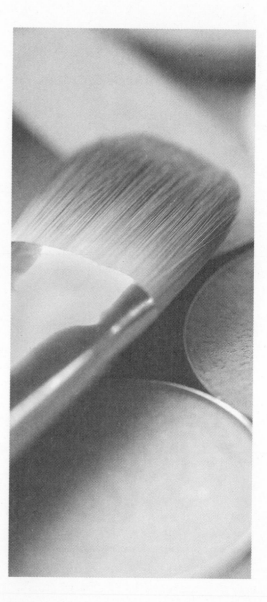

Chapter 5

Feeding your skin – beauty from within

Considering that every single skin cell on your body is maintained, repaired and even built from the materials provided in your daily diet, it is imperative that the food eaten on a regular basis is providing the nutrients needed. The skin reflects what is going on inside the body, so if there are puffiness, premature ageing, spots or even diseases, then it's time to look within and detoxify the body back to health.

Changing your diet to a more healthful one is also one of the quickest ways you can improve and beautify the skin. A healthy diet is not all bran sticks and lettuce; in fact it isn't anything like that. As a nutritionist I make it my aim to fill my body with only the best-tasting and health-giving foods available. I love eating, and my food has to look and taste gorgeous as well as making me feel and look amazing. So please do not imagine that in order to have fabulous skin you have to endure a lifetime of eating boring brown mush; I'd never eat like that, so I'm certainly not going to ask you to.

What I do suggest is that you eat plenty of super-tasty, bright and colourful, energy-giving wonder foods; this will include yummy puddings, sweet treats, chocolate shakes, ice-cream and all manner of divine dinner delights. Sounds too good to be true? Well, the proof of the healthy pudding is indeed in the eating, but before I offer you my beautifying banquet, here are some general tips for healthy skin:

MY TOP TIPS FOR FEEDING SKIN FROM WITHIN

❶ Drink two litres (two U.S. quarts) of water daily

This must be plain water – preferably filtered.

❷ Cut down on tea and coffee

Try to replace at least some of these drinks with herbal teas.

❸ Cut right down on alcohol

At the very least swap to good quality organic wines, beers and ciders, and drink in moderation (if at all). It is also wise to know your upper limits for weekly alcohol unit intake. For men this amounts to 21 units a week and for women this is 14 units per week – remember this is an upper limit, not a target to strive for. If you're not sure how many units are in your favourite drinks, ask your doctor, who may have a unit-calculator; these are useful gadgets which certainly create a shock factor when you realise how much your weekly intake really is!

❹ Be Raw-some

Try to include plenty of raw foods in your diet. If you can get your daily intake to be at least 50% raw fruits and vegetables, you will see your skin transform magically before your eyes into super-flawless beauty.

❺ Eat the rainbow

Colourful foods have the most beauty nutrients! Eat a wide variety of multi-coloured fruit and vegetables daily:

- Red – cherries, tomatoes, watermelon, grapes, red cabbage
- Orange – oranges, peppers, carrots, apricots, pumpkin
- Yellow – peppers, bananas, lemons, honeydew melon
- Green – lettuces, spinach, watercress, limes, avocado
- Blue – plums, blueberries (nope, blue Smarties do not count!)
- Purples – beetroot, aubergine, purple-sprouting broccoli, blackberries

❻ Be super

Super-foods are super nutrient-rich foods, such as avocados, brazil nuts, most berries, broccoli and lambs-lettuce, which are not only tasty but will make you glow! There are also some really exotic super-foods such as spirulina, maca, hemp powder, carob powder, powdered wheatgrass juice, raw cacao etc.

Try these powerful, health-giving plant extracts whizzed up in fresh juices and smoothies for a super health kick.

❼ Essential Fatty Acids

They are indeed 'essential' – these are the body's 'must have' fats, and they help keep the skin supple and smooth. EFAs are naturally present in most raw nuts and seeds, but you can also supplement your diet with hemp oil or linseed oil to ensure that you're getting enough. A teaspoon or two of EFA-rich plant oil in a smoothie is an easy way to add this to the diet.

❽ Sprouting

If you're thinking that eating nutritiously seems very expensive, here is the answer to super-foods on a budget – sprouts!! Not the Brussels type, but the tiny cute ones formed when you add moisture to a seed. Most of us have had mung bean sprouts at some point, but there are loads of other tastier sprouts that give you a mass of minerals and vitamins and, best of all, a packet of seeds and some jam jars cost next to nothing. Eat them with salad, in sandwiches, sprinkled on top of soups, or juice them with fruit etc. Just get those tiny nutrient factories inside your body and your skin will thank you for it.

A QUICK GUIDE TO SPROUTING

- **Get some suitable seeds – alfalfa, sunflower and mung beans are all easy to grow**
- **Place a dessertspoon full of dry seed in the bottom of a clean jam jar**
- **Fill up the jar with filtered or bottled water and leave overnight (eight hours)**
- **Next day drain the seeds leaving just a small bit of moisture in the jar**
- **Repeat twice daily for three days**
- **On day four, start eating them**
- **Store in the fridge**
- **Start a new lot of sprouts**

❾ Get nutty

Snack on small handfuls of raw nuts (brazils, almonds, hazels etc.) and seeds (sunflower, pumpkin and flax etc.) for a mineral boost and for quality proteins which will repair and maintain your skin.

❿ Feeling juicy

Nothing beats freshly made fruit and vegetable juices for a vitamin injection. Juices are digested fast, and give an instant energy and nutrient boost. Juicers are easy and cheap to pick up these days, and it's one of the best health investments you will make – keep it handy in the kitchen so daily juicing will be an easy habit to keep.

⓫ Smooth skin drinks

Smoothies are fruits whizzed up in a blender to make a thick and healthy drink. These can be very filling, and you can add powdered super-foods and EFA-rich oils to really make a health-boosting meal-in-a-glass.

As with all the advice in this book, please do not get overwhelmed. No one is asking you to suddenly turn into Miss super-sprouter-juicer-organic-clothing-wearer-teetotal-health-freak. These are just suggestions that you can pick and choose from; in fact implementing just one of the steps above will give you noticeable results.

Now before we move on to the tasty recipes, here are some foods to be wary of, as they are often considered, by holistic nutritionists, to be anti-nutrients – foods which actually destroy the nutrients in the body rather than provide them.

MY WORST FIVE ANTI-NUTRIENT FOODS

❶ Sugar

Number one anti-nutrient – this means white sugar, brown sugar, molasses and yes even honey to some extent. In fact any sugar which has been extracted from its original form is a liability for the body, not just stripping out the nutrients but also suppressing immunity too. Sugar in its natural form (i.e. wrapped up in a fibrous raw fruit or vegetable) is fine and provides the body with needed energy, but the pure stuff just provides empty calories.

❷ Salt

Similarly, natural mineral salts present in raw fruits and vegetables do not present a problem, but adding extracted salt to food is messing with the natural balance in the body. Too much salt will result in puffy skin as well as a whole host of other health issues.

❸ Fried fatty foods

As if the food wasn't fatty enough, it gets heated in grease too. Heated fats and oils clog up the body and also prevent the assimilation of the essential fatty acids which are necessary for skin health. Be aware of your body – does it feel healthy after eating a fry-up?

❹ Alcohol

We are a nation of binge-drinkers, it seems, and it is playing havoc with our looks! Alcohol is very dehydrating to the whole body as well as the skin – keep on boozing if you want saggy, dry, sallow skin!

❺ Junk/processed foods

They taste horrid and are always way too high in bad fats, salt and sugar. They should be avoided at all costs if possible. The body cannot build healthy skin from junk materials.

It is important not to get too hung up about your dietary intake and become obsessive; a healthy body is more resilient and so can cope better when you have the occasional junky food or lavish cocktail. Concentrate on getting 80% of your diet healthy and do not worry too much about the other 20% for now. Be gentle with yourself and give yourself time to make changes; this way any changes made are more likely to stick and you will reap the long-term health benefits.

One of the ways you can make changes is to do it on a meal-by-meal basis, starting with breakfast. Once the healthy breakfast habit is totally formed, then (and only then) move on to lunch and make changes there, and so on. After a few months your entire diet will have improved dramatically, yet you will have barely noticed. This 'health by stealth' approach really works for long-term dietary change.

The following food section is really just a 'taster' to get you started on the healthy skin path; for more in-depth information refer to the recipe books in the *Resources* section, or alternatively, if you are very serious about changing your diet, seek out a local holistic nutritionist or naturopath who will work with you and help you to adjust to a new healthier way of eating which can be life-changing!

A HEALTHY START TO THE MORNING

This is the best health habit to start implementing; when breakfast is firing up the body with quality energy and nutrients, you'll be well on your way to feeling super-gorgeous and glowingly beautiful every day. Once this healthy-breakfast habit is formed, that's one third of the diet changed already! How easy is that?

The very best food you can eat in the morning is fruit; this provides plenty of slow-release energy plus all those wonderful skin-glowing vitamins and antioxidants. Not only is fruit mega-healthy, but it's surely the tastiest health food on the planet! As much as I love chocolate cake, I'd much rather munch on a watermelon or guzzle on a fresh ripe peach. Don't worry that you won't be full enough – the recipes below will leave you satisfied enough to ignore the coffee-break doughnuts. Plus, considering that you can't really get fat from eating fruit, you can eat as much as you want while you adjust to this lighter breakfast – you're not 'on a diet', so don't suffer or go hungry for the sake of beauty.

You can also add a teaspoon of hemp oil (or other EFA-rich oil) and a teaspoon of super-food powder (spirulina etc.) to these breakfasts to boost their nutritional power even more.

A super smoothie for those in a hurry.

Breakfast in a glass (vegan)

Ingredients
- 1 large ripe organic banana
- 1 handful organic raisins
- 1 small handful organic porridge oats
- 300-500ml/½-1 pint filtered water
- Shake of powdered cinnamon
- Dash of vanilla essence (optional)

How to make
- The night before, place the oats and raisins in 300ml/½ pint of water
- In the morning place the mixture in a blender
- Add the banana and spice
- Blend thoroughly
- Add more water if necessary

- Drink within half an hour; feel this yummy breakfast satisfy you completely

Choccy banana dream shake (vegan)

One for the chocoholics.

Ingredients

- 2 organic bananas
- 1 handful organic dried dates
- 1 tablespoon of raw cocoa powder (or raw carob powder)
- Quarter of a vanilla pod
- 300-500ml/½-1 pint filtered water

How to make

- Soak the dates overnight in 300ml/10 fl oz of water
- In the morning blend everything together
- Add more water if necessary
- Drink it within half an hour and enjoy the hit of the nutritious chocolate

Deluxe fruit salad (vegan)

Refreshing and juicy.

Ingredients

- 2 plums
- 1 ripe pear
- 7 strawberries
- 1 tablespoon blueberries
- Half a pink grapefruit

How to make

- Chop the pear and plums into chunks
- Halve the strawberries
- Mix up in a bowl with the whole blueberries
- Squeeze the pink grapefruit juice over the fruit
- Eat with the eyes closed and enjoy the tangy sensations

Winter apple porridge (vegan)

This is so warming on a cold day. The apples add sweetness, so there's no need to add sugar!

Ingredients

- 1 cup organic porridge oats
- 2 cups filtered water
- 2 small (or 1 large) organic apples
- Dash of cinnamon (optional)

How to make

- Put the oats and water into a pan on low heat
- Peel and chop the apples
- Add the apples to the pan once the porridge is simmering
- Stir frequently and add more water if necessary

- Once oats are cooked and apples soft, mash it up with a potato masher
- Eat while warm

Tropical morning

This is so dreamy and creamy; imagine you're on a sunny island in a hammock.

Ingredients
- Half a tin of organic coconut milk
- 1 organic banana
- 1 ripe organic mango
- 1 organic lime

How to make
- Chop the banana and mango
- Put in a blender with the coconut milk
- Add the juice and grated zest from the lime
- Blend thoroughly until smooth
- Sit outside in the sun and drink slowly

LUSH LUNCHES AND DELISH DINNERS

So now you've got all those tasty breakfasts to enjoy, here are some delicious ideas for a skin-feeding lunch. I've offered recipes that are all suitable for eating at work, so there's no excuse for not taking a healthy packed lunch. When your colleagues notice how gorgeous your skin is and how much younger you're starting to look, they'll all be wanting to eat what you bring in. These dishes are also great for dinner-time too. It is better to eat lightly at the end of the day, as stodgy heavy meals can make the body and mind lethargic.

The great thing with eating this way is that because all the foods are so healthy it doesn't matter if you just want a pudding for dinner or just a smoothie for lunch, you'll still be packing the body full of vital nutrients which will make you glow inside and out. You may have noticed that most of these foods are raw. This is no accident: raw foods are the best building materials for the body, and by eating at least 50% of your diet raw you can be sure that beautiful skin and super-health are easily achievable right now.

Chips and dips (vegan)

The healthy version.

Ingredients
For the chips
- 2 organic wholemeal pitta breads

How to make
- Slice the pittas into diagonal strips
- Then cut across the strips to make diamond/square shapes
- Pull the two halves of the bread shapes apart
- Place on a baking tray and put in a medium oven for 10 minutes

- Move the chips about, then put back in oven for a further 10 minutes
- Check frequently as some will crisp up more quickly than others
- Remove when brown and crispy
- Leave to cool

Guacamole (vegan)

This is yummy, green and full of vitamin E for healthy skin

Ingredients
- 1 ripe organic Hass avocado
- 1 organic tomato
- Half a fresh mild chilli
- 1 clove garlic
- Juice of 2 limes
- A small handful fresh coriander stalks

How to make
- Halve the avocado and scoop out the flesh
- Put everything into a food processor
- Process until creamy but not overly smooth
- Serve with pitta chips and crudités (carrot sticks, cucumber slices etc.)

Beany feast (vegan)

A really filling tasty dip.

Ingredients
- 1 tin organic butter beans
- 2 cloves organic garlic
- Juice of 2 organic lemons
- A dash of organic olive oil

How to make
- Drain off the beans and rinse under running water
- Place everything into a blender
- Whiz up until smooth and creamy
- Serve with pitta chips and crudités (carrot sticks, cucumber slices etc.)

Salad sticks (vegan)

I love these; they look so cute and are delicious.

Ingredients
A combination of any of the following:
- Organic cherry tomatoes
- Organic stoned olives
- Chunks of organic cucumber
- Chunks of organic peppers
- Organic raw mushrooms
- Organic grapes
- Fresh basil leaves

How to make
- Fill up wooden skewers with a mix of these foods
- Eat as they are or serve with guacamole etc.

Cabbage wraps (vegan)

These are as tasty and filling as the usual kind of wrap sandwich, but being wheat-free they don't leave you bloated and sleepy afterwards.

Ingredients
- Several leaves from a soft cabbage (the pointy ones are the best)
- Some of the 'Beany feast' dip (see p.36)
- Shredded lettuce
- Grated carrot
- Grated beetroot

How to make
- Spread a thick layer of beany dip on a cabbage leaf
- Sprinkle a thick layer of salady bits in a line down the middle of the leaf on top of the dip
- Roll up the cabbage leaf tightly like a tortilla wrap sandwich
- Secure with a cocktail stick if necessary
- Eat straight away or wrap in greaseproof paper to eat later

PUDDINGS FOR PERFECT SKIN

Here is the really exciting bit: all those yummy desserts that are normally frowned on when trying to eat a better diet – well, here are gorgeous puds that are good for you, so eat up and have second helpings even (nutritionist's orders!).

Chocolate mousse (vegan)

You won't believe that this is a health food, it just tastes so naughty!

Ingredients
- 1 ripe organic avocado (the smooth Fuerte type are good as they have little taste)
- 1 ripe organic banana
- 1 tablespoon raw cocoa powder or raw carob powder
- Dash of vanilla essence

How to make
- Blend all together in a food processor or mouli
- Decorate with a physalis fruit for style
- Add a dash of orange juice or fresh mint for a variation

Sexy ice-cream (vegan)

Shut your eyes and melt into this silky smooth treat:

Ingredients
- 3 ripe organic bananas
- Half a vanilla pod

How to make
- Slice and freeze the bananas overnight
- Scrape out the seeds of the vanilla pod and add to the sliced bananas
- Blend in a food processor until the consistency of soft ice-cream
- Variation: add other frozen fruit, e.g. strawberries or blackberries

Banoffee pie (vegan)

Yes, there's even a healthy version of this!

Ingredients
- 100g/3½ oz brazil nuts
- 200g/7 oz dried dates
- 3 ripe organic bananas
- 100-300ml/3½-10 fl oz organic coconut milk

How to make
- Soak 100g/3½ oz dried dates overnight in 100ml/6¾ tbsp coconut milk
- Put the nuts and rest of the dried dates in a food processor and blend to make a sticky dough
- Press the 'dough' into a small tart tin and refrigerate for a few hours
- Blend the coconut milk/soaked date mixture to make a fudgey sauce
- Add more coconut milk if necessary
- Layer sliced bananas and fudgey sauce in the nut/date base
- Finish with a covering of sauce on top
- Share with friends – it's rich

QUICK TREATS

Salads

Salads from fresh organic ripe fruits are always nice. Try:
- Sliced apple, blackberries and plums
- Sliced mango, sliced papaya and passion fruit
- Watermelon chunks, honeydew melon chunks and Piel de Sapo melon chunks
- Halved strawberries, raspberries and halved red grapes

Smoothies

Easy to make and eat:
- Blend one chopped mango with juice from three oranges
- Blend raspberries with the juice from three blood oranges

- Blend one banana with a punnet of strawberries
- Blend ten strawberries with half a cucumber and fresh mint leaves
- Blend a whole honeydew melon

This chapter has given you a taster of the sort of super-healthy snacks and dishes that can be enjoyed in the pursuit of health, vitality and beautiful skin. Try these tasty recipes on a daily basis and you'll be amazed at how your skin will improve and how good you will feel. The skincare-potion recipes are awesome, but even they need the back-up of a healthy diet in order to really make a difference.

Feed your skin, from outside and in.

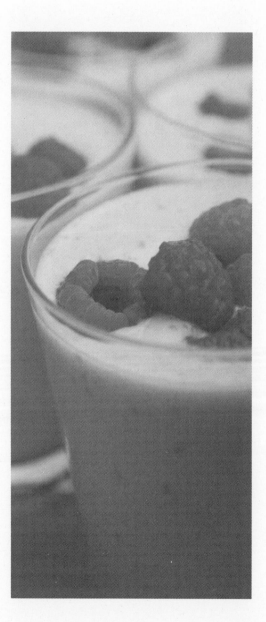

Chapter 6

Potion-making basics

This chapter covers all the basic information you need before embarking on your newly discovered skill of 'potion-making': health and safety, the ingredients, equipment, techniques, and packaging, and what to do if it turns out wrong!

Please familiarise yourself with the Health and Safety section (next column) as there are important issues raised there; if you are pregnant or suffer from allergies, this information is particularly important, as you will need to know which ingredients and essential oils to avoid.

There is also lots to learn by way of techniques, equipment used, and even a breakdown of the ingredients. Many of this may be unfamiliar to you, so here's your chance to really learn and prepare for the fun stuff. Don't let any of the odd-sounding ingredients put you off – some of them may seem strange and entirely foreign, but they are all readily available from the suppliers listed in the *Resources* section. Most of the ingredients are very economical to buy and many of them will be in your kitchen cupboards already.

This is also true of the equipment, most of which you will already own, as potion-making tends to require the same bits and pieces as cooking. So, generally speaking, apart from some of the more exotic ingredients, many of you will already be well equipped for making your own unique holistic cosmetics straight away.

HEALTH AND SAFETY

1 Never eat/drink your potions (even though they may look tasty!).

2 Make sure your hands are dry before using potions – added water will encourage bacterial contamination.

3 Always store potions and ingredients in a dry, cool place out of direct sunlight.

4 Potion-making can be messy, so tie up your hair and wear an apron.

5 Always wash your hands before making and using potions.

6 Make sure your containers are scrupulously clean and dry before using.

7 Never 'water down' a potion to get the last bit out.

8 Consult your midwife before using any essential oils in pregnancy and see advice on the NHS Direct website **www.nhsdirect.nhs.uk;** make sure your aromatherapy practitioner is qualified – see: **www.aromatherapycouncil.co.uk**

9 There are currently no 100% natural

preservatives which work as effectively as the chemical ones, so please store your potions in accordance with the instructions, always label them with the date made, and do not exceed their given shelf-life. If in doubt, chuck it out! (on the compost heap).

⑩ Any individual can be allergic to even the most benign of natural ingredients. Please do a patch test before using any ingredient or concoction in this book.

How to do a patch test:

- Clean and dry the crook of the elbow
- Place a small amount of ingredient or potion there
- Cover with a lint-free dressing
- Leave for 24 hours
- Check for a reaction, and if there is one, avoid that substance

INGREDIENTS

Just as a cook will always have certain staples to hand, so it is with potion-making. Here are the skincare product staples:

Plant fats/butters

These are the solid fats extracted from certain tropical plants; these are used for solid products such as body bars and melts, as well as used to form moisturisers and creams.

The most common ones are:

- Cocoa butter – a chocolate-scented butter
- Shea butter – a sticky fat from a Ghanaian tree
- Coconut butter – an almost liquid fat from coconuts
- Mango butter – a scentless white fat from mango pips

Plant oils

These are the liquid fats extracted from certain plants; look out for the cold-pressed varieties as they will be more nutritious for the skin. The oils are used to dilute essential oils and are also blended with the solid butters to make creams and moisturisers.

The most commonly used ones are:

- Almond oil – a very light and almost odourless oil, ideal for all skin types
- Apricot oil – another all-purpose light oil
- Avocado oil – a rich nourishing oil for dry or mature skins
- Sunflower oil – an all-purpose oil, often used for macerating
- Jojoba oil – a rich waxy oil which is almost identical to the sebum that our skin produces

Macerated oils

These are plant oils which have had medicinal herbs or scented flowers steeped in them.

These are easily made at home, and some common ones are:

- Calendula oil – from marigold petals, useful for sensitive skins

- Rose oil – wonderfully soothing and great for dry and mature skin

- Carrot oil – full of beta-carotene, very healing for problem skin

- Monoi de Tahiti – an exotically fragrant oil for massage and beauty

Essential oils

Concentrated aromatic essences, distilled from certain plants. They are used for their medicinal qualities as well as their scent.

Common cosmetic ones are:

- Rose – for rejuvenating mature skin

- Lavender – cleansing and healing properties

- Chamomile – very healing and soothing for sensitive skin

- Geranium – tones and brightens the skin

- Lemon, lime or orange – great flavours for lip-balms etc

- Rosemary – for hair-care

Flower waters/distillates

Also known as Hydrosols or Hydrolats, these scented waters are the by-product of the distillation of essential oils. They are used as the watery part of moisturisers, as well as for deodorants, facial toners and to simply freshen up the face on a hot day.

Common cosmetic ones are:

- Rosewater – sweetly smelling and gorgeous in facial products

- Orange flower water – used as a facial toner, it smells like an orange grove

- Peppermint water – so refreshing to splash on the feet or as a mouthwash

- Lavender water – useful to soothe troubled skin

Herbs/flowers

The 'active ingredients' of any beauty product. So many herbs, so little time! They are used whole in bath products, ground in skin scrubs and are also made into infusions (tea).

The common ones are:

- Lavender – used for centuries for cleansing and soothing skin; brilliant for burns

- Rose petals – a soft soothing herb suitable for all skins, especially dry and mature ones

- Chamomile – used medicinally for eczema and other skin conditions

- Calendula – a well-known medicinal herb used for skin conditions
- Vanilla – this sweetly scented pod is used particularly for its perfume
- Rosemary – use for cleansing, hair-care and soothing muscles
- Soapwort – a natural shampoo plant

Kitchen edibles

- Oats – used for washing, skin-scrubbing, and soothing sensitive skin
- Beans/nuts – ground into gritty powders for skin-scrubs
- Yoghurt – used in face-masks
- Fruit – used in face and body masks
- Cocoa/chocolate – used for luxurious body treats
- Sea salt – used in bath salts, dental care and body-scrubs
- Sugar – use for body-scrubs
- Bicarbonate of soda – for explosive bath bombs, dental care and deodorants
- Citric acid – mixed with bicarbonate of soda for bath bombs
- Citrus peels – used for-skin scrubs and scenting oils
- Honey – sticky sugar from bees which makes soothing face-masks and scrubs

Miscellaneous bits

- Green clay – used for refining face-masks
- Rhassoul mud – used for deep cleansing and hair-care
- Irish Moss – a gelatinous seaweed used for hair-care and detoxifying body-packs
- Gum tragacanth – a plant gum which is a natural emulsifier
- Beeswax – used to thicken and emulsify creams and herbal salves
- Glycerine – a by-product of saponifying plant oils for soap; a good moisturiser and natural preservative

All of the ingredients listed above can be easily obtained from the suppliers listed in the back of this book (p.170).

EQUIPMENT

As mentioned before, potion-making is really just like cooking, so most of the bits listed below will be familiar. It is definitely a good idea to buy separate equipment if you'll be doing a lot of potion-making, as it stops cross-contamination. Let's face it – nobody wants garlic-scented face-cream! All the equipment listed below is available in good cook shops.

Knives

A palette knife for transferring potions to pots, and sharp knives for chopping.

Heatproof bowls

Glass or enamel, for mixing and using as a bain-marie.

Chopping-board

For chopping plant fats and other hard ingredients.

Whisks and mini-whisks

Big ones for whipping up large butters, small ones for lip-balms etc.

Stirrers

I prefer to use wooden sticks like chopsticks or cocktail sticks to stir my mixtures.

Wooden spoons

For mixing batches of dry goods etc.

Cheese-grater

For grating citrus peels and cocoa butter.

Measuring jugs

Big ones for pints etc., and smaller ones for measuring 100ml/6¾ tbsp and less.

Sieve

For straining macerated oils.

Moulds

Ice-cube trays are fab for melts, soap moulds or mini cake tins for massage bars.

Bain-marie

A heatproof bowl set over a pan of simmering water to melt fats gently.

Coffee grinder

For grinding dried herbs, flowers, nuts and pulses. Can be electric or manual.

Pestle and mortar

For bruising fresh herbs and grinding dried goods. Also for creaming up shea butter if you don't have a food processor.

Weighing scales

Digital ones that can measure as low as 1g are ideal.

Food processor

For whipping up creamy body butters and moisturisers.

Slow cooker (non-essential)

For macerating oils/fats easily.

Cider press (non-essential)

For pressing out large quantities of macerated oils.

TECHNIQUES

Preparing fresh herbs

If you grow your own herbs and flowers, they can be used fresh to make macerated oils – see Chapter 3 (p.20) *Essential oils* for making these – or you can dry them out to be used in any of the recipes calling for dried herbs. You can also dry your own fruit peels to use in potions too.

Always pick your herb or flower on a dry morning after the dew has dried.

To dry herbs:

• Hang bunches of herbs upside down in a warm place for a week or so until they feel crispy

• Carefully remove the dried leaves and/or flowering tops

• Discard the stems

• Rub the dried herbs between clean hands until roughly crumbled

• Store in a clean dry glass jar

• Label with the date and do not store for longer than 12 months

To dry individual flowers (e.g. calendula) or petals (e.g. rose)

• Place petals or flower heads on sheets of organic kitchen-towel roll on a tray

• Place somewhere dry and warm – an airing cupboard is ideal

• Turn the flowers and petals daily until dry and crispy to touch

• Store in a glass jar and label; do not store for longer than 12 months

To dry citrus peels

• Peel an orange (or lemon, lime etc.)

• Eat the orange!

• Place the peel on a sheet of organic kitchen paper on a tray

• Place somewhere dry and warm (e.g. the airing cupboard)

• Turn the peels daily until dry and crispy to touch

• Store in a glass jar and label; do not store for longer than 12 months

Grinding

Some recipes call for the herb or flower to be powdered; this is done easily in a coffee grinder. Some ingredients are available in powdered form from some suppliers.

Infusing

A herbal infusion is basically a herbal tea, so you can even use a bought tea-bag (for example, if a recipe calls for nettle infusion – just make nettle tea). The general rule is

25 g /1 oz of fresh or dried herb to 500ml /1 pint of boiling water.

Macerating

This is the steeping of herbs in a plant oil to extract the scent and/or medicinal properties. Maceration is covered in depth in Chapter 3, *Essential oils* (p.20).

Blending

This is simply mixing or whisking to bring all the ingredients together in one uniform concoction – like making a cake-mix!

Grating

Some recipes call for grated plant butters or fresh citrus peel. Always use the finer grating side of a normal cheese-grater.

Melting

This is always done in a bain-marie (see section on Equipment, p.44) as the delicate plant fats melt very easily and they can overheat and start to cook if just melted in a normal pan. It is also possible to melt fats gently on one of those candle-powered plate-warmer gadgets you see in Indian restaurants.

Straining

When straining off fats after macerating herbs, it can be hard to get all the bits out completely. The best way is to strain through a normal sieve, then strain again through a sieve that is lined with muslin. If the oil is still bitty, a final straining through a funnel lined with a coffee filter paper should do it.

PACKAGING

In the spirit of being planet-friendly it makes sense to package our wonderful organic eco-concoctions in suitable environmentally-sound packaging. There are many options to choose from, and most are very low-cost or even free; there are even some funky gift-packaging ideas for you to choose from (see p.47).

When reusing bottles and jars, it is important to make sure they are really clean and dry before use. Wash them in hot soapy water using a bottle brush for hard to reach places, rinse in cold clean water, then place upside-down on a clean baking tray and place somewhere warm (Aga top, airing cupboard or even the bottom of a very low-heat oven) until bone dry. Store in ziplock or similar bags until needed.

Glass

This is the best material to put your lotions and potions into as it is inert and therefore will not taint your products, and glass is easy to clean and reuse too. Collect up old potion bottles and jars from friends – most people have some pretty bottles stashed away.

Ask chip shops for their old pickled egg display jars; most are only too happy to get rid of them and they make brilliant storage containers for bulk-bought dried herbs.

Hotels will often save you the mini jam jars that they use at breakfasts, which is a great way to end up with hundreds of lip-balm pots and mini potion jars.

Cloth

Scraps of old natural fabric and ribbon can be sewn into simple drawstring bags to contain bath melts, massage bars, bath salts etc. If you're feeling extravagant then purchase a small amount of new organic cotton or hemp. For those who are handy with a needle, decorate your bags with embroidery, appliqué or beadwork for a stunning potion pouch.

Paper

Recycled, hand-made and even plain 'common-or-garden' brown baking parchment can be used to attractively wrap massage bars, melts and solid scrub bars. Use raffia, ribbon, dried herbs and your imagination for a gorgeous eco-packaging solution.

Cardboard boxes

Save up pretty gift boxes in all shapes and sizes to make boxed-sets of potions. If plain, these can be decorated artistically.

Baskets

These can be found in all shapes and sizes, in second-hand shops as well as new. They make lovely receptacles to arrange a pretty potion display.

Gift ideas

Here are a few ideas to get you started:

- Arrange a jar of hand scrub, hand-balm and a nail-brush inside a terracotta flower-pot for a gorgeous gardener's gift set

- Make-up a selection of herbal bath tea blends (dried herbs and flowers in mini muslin bags) and arrange inside a second-hand china teapot

- Roll up a solid face-scrub or mask sushi-style in sheets of nori seaweed, and present in a Japanese bamboo dish

- A variety of different bath melts look cute inside an old-fashioned glass sweetie jar. Throw in a handful of scented rosebuds to complete the look

The recipes

So now you've heard every reason under the sun to avoid toxic toiletries and to make your own natural ones instead, here are the recipes – a multitude of miraculous and marvellous mixtures to soothe, nourish, cleanse and tone.

There are:

- Facials to beautify

- Bath treats for pampering
- Love potions for romance
- Body butters for bliss
- Babycare potions for eco-kids

Let us grasp the whisk of dermal destiny and step into a world of scented decadence, where rose petals fall from the sky into a sea of vanilla pod-infused melted cocoa butter.

WHEN POTIONS GO WRONG!

It's hard to go wrong with potion-making, as most mixtures can be re-melted and remade with an adjustment of solids and liquids. If something seems unfixable, just rename it, e.g.:

- **A too-liquid moisturiser becomes a lotion**
- **A too-hard face-cream becomes a lip-balm**
- **A very hard moisturiser is a bath melt**
- **A strong-smelling macerated oil becomes a medicinal ointment**
- **A very stiff face-scrub becomes fragrant bathing grains**
- **Anything mouldy becomes compost!**

chapter seven
the face

Cleansers

Our face is usually the first thing people notice about us; smooth skin and sparkly eyes speak volumes about our health and beauty. Unfortunately, most of us tend to hide the state of our skin or our natural beauty by plastering on lots of make-up. Not only is this make-up itself usually toxic to the skin, but it covers our natural looks. On top of all that, the chances are that we started the day by washing then moisturising with a variety of toxic skin-pollutants.

It's time to really feed our faces with gorgeous hand-made potions filled with delightful nature-given ingredients that will nourish our skin and make our faces truly healthy and glowing!

CLEANSERS

With regard to facial cleansing, it is preferable to use the mechanical action of gentle massage and scrubbing with natural exfoliant, than to use the grease-binding chemical action of detergents or soap. Used on moistened skin with a gentle massaging action, skin-scrubs will clean without destroying your natural oils, leaving your face soft and clean but not tight and dry. It is also possible to use oils and butters to cleanse; these work on greasy dirt and make-up very well.

Fairy face-scrub

Shelf-life: 2 months
Skin types: all

A sweetly scented and gently exfoliating cleanser, which is great for all skin types but particularly soothing for sensitive skins.

Ingredients

- 2 tablespoons ground almonds
- 1 tablespoon fine oatmeal
- 3-5 teaspoons powdered dried rose petals
- 3-5 teaspoons powdered dried orange peel
- 3-5 teaspoons powdered dried lavender flowers
- 3-5 teaspoons finely grated cocoa butter
- 1 tablespoon mango butter or coconut fat, roughly chopped
- 1-3 teaspoons almond oil

How to make

- Put your ground almonds and oatmeal into a mixing bowl. Run the dried flowers and peel through a coffee grinder, or use a pestle and mortar to powder.
- Add the powder to the bowl.
- Grate chunk of cocoa butter into the bowl.
- Stir to mix it up.
- Add the chopped plant fat and almond oil.
- Mix and rub together until you have a stiff paste.
- Squish the mixture firmly into a nice glass jar.

That's it!

How to use

Firstly splash some warm water on your face, then dig out a walnut-sized lump of the gorgeously scented mixture, squish it in your moist hands for a second just to make it spreadable, then gently massage onto your face and rinse off when done. Your face will be glowing and as soft as a rose petal.

Sunshine face butter

Shelf-life: 6 months
Skin types: great for dry and sensitive skins

This creamy cleanser uses soothing marigold (*Calendula officinalis*), which is a bright orange daisy-like flower used medicinally for troubled and sensitive skins. The calendula oil is a macerated oil (whereby a medicinal plant is steeped in a plant oil for up to a month to extract the herbal properties). Macerated oils can be easily made at home or bought from an aromatherapy supplier.

How to make

- In the bain-marie, melt together 100ml/6¾ tbsp of calendula oil and 65g/2¼ oz of cocoa butter
- Once melted, turn off the heat and carefully remove the bowl
- Continuously stir the blend until it starts thickening and cooling; whip with the mini-whisk until thick and creamy
- Add 20 drops of each essential oil
- Decant your creamy cleansing balm to a glass jar and label

NB. You can easily adjust this mixture to the consistency you desire: if you want it to be thicker, re-melt with extra cocoa butter; if you desire a runnier lotion, re-melt with more oil.

How to use

Massage a generous amount onto the face, and then, using a square of muslin or flannel and hot water, gently remove the balm. Your face will be beautifully clean and smelling gorgeous too.

Ingredients

- 100ml/6¾ tbsp calendula oil
- 65g/2¼ oz cocoa butter, roughly chopped
- 20 drops sweet orange
- 20 drops mandarin essential oil

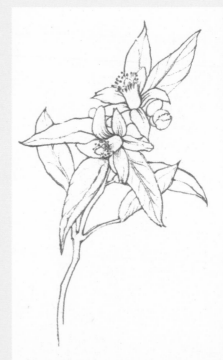

Orange

Washing grains

Shelf-life: 6 months
Skin types: suitable for all but very sensitive skin

Ingredients

- 100g/3½ oz dried whole adzuki beans
- Scented grains – add 50g/1¾ oz dried lavender or rose petals to the beans in the grinder
- Fruity grains – add 50g/1¾ oz dried citrus peel (lime is great for men) to the beans in the grinder
- Spicy grains – add 25g/1 oz ground cinnamon or ginger to the ground beans

For him – add:

- 20g/¾ oz dried lime peel
- 20g/¾ oz dried bay leaves
- 10g/⅜ oz allspice per 100g/3½ oz of beans

For her – add:

- 30g/1 oz dried rose petals
- 30g/1 oz orris-root powder
- 1 inch piece of fresh vanilla pod per 100g/3½ oz of beans

This warm and silky blend will gently scent and polish. A very well-known skincare company used to sell something very similar, but it was rather expensive – here is an improved version which will cost hardly anything! Adzuki beans can be found in most supermarkets and health stores.

How to make

- Grind up the beans into a gritty powder in a coffee grinder
- Powder the chosen herb/spice blend in the coffee grinder
- Blend the mixture well in a mixing bowl
- Store in a pretty glass jar

How to use

Wet the skin and pour a little powder into a moist hand. Gently massage the fine grains over the face and rinse.

Ultra-cleansing oil

Shelf-life: 12 months
Skin types: suitable for all

It may sound odd to use an oil to clean the skin; however, oil is excellent at removing greasy dirt and make-up from the skin as it acts like a solvent into which grime dissolves, and this can then be easily wiped away. In fact, I've never found anything better for removing really tough eye make-up and mascara.

This blend uses jojoba oil because it is almost identical to the skin's own natural oil (sebum) and so really works in tune with your skin to dissolve grime and greasy dirt.

Ingredients

- 50ml/3½ tbsp jojoba
- 25ml/5 tsp sweet almond oil
- 25ml/5 tsp apricot oil
- 10 drops geranium essential oil
- 10 drops lemon essential oil

How to make

- Blend the plant oils in a measuring jug
- Add the essential oils
- Stir gently but thoroughly to blend the oils
- Pour into a nice glass bottle

How to use

Warm a small amount of the cleansing oil in your hands, then use light stroking motions to gently massage the oil into the skin. Leave for a few seconds then, using either an organic cotton-wool pad or moist warm cloth, gently remove the oil. This will leave skin fresh, glowing and delightfully scented.

Toners

Toners are basically refreshing liquids that are spritzed onto the face. They are often used to remove the last traces of a cleanser before moisturising, but they can also be used just to freshen up the face and to set finished make-up. Commercial toners often use alcohol, which is very astringent and will dry out the skin; the following recipes are based on flower waters, which are lightly scented and gentle. Toners are also great to help remove face-masks and face-packs which are being a bit stubborn.

Rosy Refresher

Shelf-life: 3 months
Skin types: suitable for all, but great for dry and mature skins

This fragrant flowery toner is great for dry or mature skins; frankincense has long been used in anti-ageing formulas because of its preservative qualities. Gentle rose is wonderfully softening, and has an amazing smell.

Ingredients

- 50ml/3½ tbsp rosewater
- 50ml/3½ tbsp frankincense water
- 50ml/3½ tbsp geranium water

How to make

- Pour equal amounts of each flower water into a jug
- Stir until well blended
- Using a funnel, pour into the bottle and label

How to use

As a face refresher, simply spritz over the face as needed. If using as a toner, soak two cotton pads with the solution and wipe gently over the face after cleansing and before using a moisturiser.

Gentle herbal spritz

Shelf-life: 3 months
Skin types: suitable for all, but great for sensitive skins

Ingredients

- 50ml/3½ tbsp rosewater
- 50ml/3½ tbsp lavender water
- 50ml/3½ tbsp chamomile water

This toner contains gentle soothing herbs which makes it ideal for sensitive or troubled skin.

How to make

- Pour equal amounts of each flower water into a jug
- Stir until well blended
- Using a funnel, pour into a bottle and label

How to use

As a face refresher, simply spritz over the face as needed. If using as a toner, soak two cotton pads with the solution and wipe gently over the face after cleansing and before using a moisturiser.

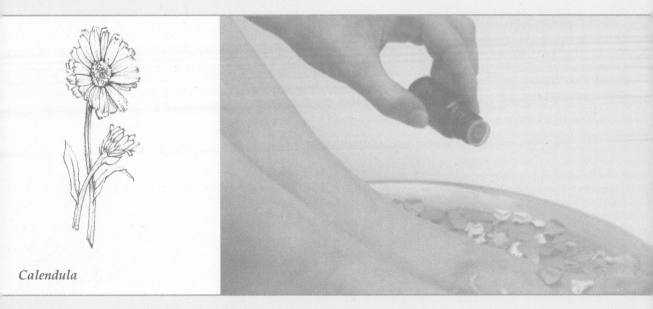

Calendula

Citrusy spritz

Shelf-life: 3 months
Skin types: good for oily skins

A zesty toner for oily skins, containing uplifting lemon balm and spicy juniper for controlling shine without drying the skin out.

How to make

- Pour equal amounts of each flower water into a jug
- Stir until well blended
- Using the funnel, pour into the bottle and label

How to use

As a face refresher, simply spritz over the face as needed. If using as a toner, soak two cotton pads with the solution and wipe gently over the face after cleansing and before using a moisturiser.

Ingredients

- 50ml/3½ tbsp lemon balm water
- 50ml/3½ tbsp orange flower water
- 50ml/3½ tbsp orange peel water
- 50ml/3½ tbsp juniper water

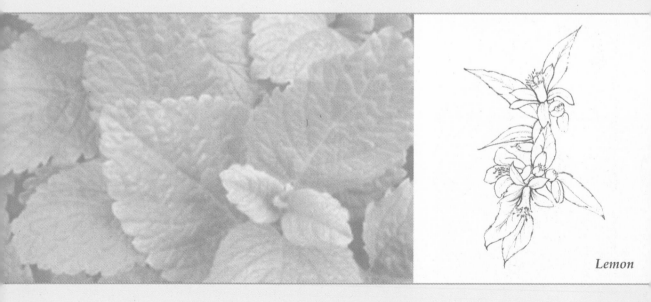

Lemon

Skin–balancing mist

Shelf-life: 3 months
Skin types: suitable for all

Ingredients

- 50ml/3½ tbsp geranium water
- 50ml/3½ tbsp clary sage water
- 50ml/3½ tbsp rosewater

This is a recipe containing plants that really help to tone up the skin and balance out any skin problems. It has a lovely smell too.

How to make

- Pour equal amounts of each flower water into a jug
- Stir until well blended
- Using the funnel, pour into a bottle and label

How to use

As a face refresher, simply spritz over the face as needed. If using as a toner, soak two cotton pads with the solution and wipe gently over the face after cleansing and before using a moisturiser.

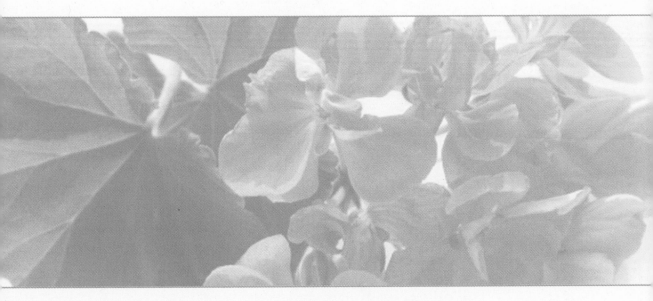

Moisturisers

So what is a 'moisturiser' exactly? Generally speaking, it refers to a creamy gloop consisting primarily of emulsified fat or oil and water. This emulsion is designed to re-hydrate the skin (to 'moisturise' it) and also to make it feel nice and soft after cleansing, by coating the skin in a layer of emollient oils or fats. Most commercial moisturisers contain petro-chemical by-products, animal fats and alcohol (as well as other rubbish). Outlandish claims are often made for the rejuvenating and beautifying properties of these man-made mixtures; unfortunately this is simply marketing hype.

Even the term 'moisturiser' is a bit misleading, as the skin can only be fed and hydrated from the inside, by having a natural and water-sufficient diet. It cannot be 'moisture-ised' by applying water to its surface – if it could, then sitting in a bath would quench thirst!

This means, therefore, that a moisturising cream does not need to contain any water at all; it just needs to be able to feed the skin and make it beautifully silky after washing. Simple plant oils and butters are excellent emollients to nourish and soothe. Making a 100% natural moisturiser from scratch may seem like a daunting task, but it is quite simple, and as easy as making a cake.

Whipped shea cream

Shelf-life: 6 months
Skin types: suitable for all

Ingredients

- 50g/1¾ oz fair-trade shea butter
- 50-100ml/3½-6¾ tbsp organic sweet almond oil

Optional essential oils:

- 30 drops Neroli
- 15 drops orange
- 15 drops tangerine

This is a very simple plain face-cream to make. It can be customised by adding essential oils to make a therapeutic potion or scented balm. Shea butter comes from West Africa, where it is traditionally gathered by women and is a renowned skin food and sun protector.

How to make

- Pound the shea butter in the pestle and mortar until smooth
- Gradually trickle in the oil while mixing
- Stop when it looks white and soft like semi-molten ice-cream
- At this point, whip with a mini-whisk to really fluff it up
- Using a palette knife, scrape the fluffy gloop into a jar, add the lid and label

How to use

After washing and removing make-up, take a small amount and massage gently onto face and neck daily.

Creamy cocoa butter

Shelf-life: 6 months
Skin type: suitable for all

This is a similar recipe to Whipped shea cream on the previous page, but uses deliciously chocolate-scented cocoa butter instead. Unlike shea butter, cocoa butter can be purchased completely raw (cold-pressed) so that all the nutrients are present and it can really feed your skin. Because it melts at a low 37 °C (98°F), it starts to work the minute it touches the face.

How to make

- Chop up the solid cocoa butter
- Place in a bain-marie on very low heat until it just becomes liquid
- Add half the almond oil, mix and remove from the heat
- Let it cool to a fudgey mix, but don't let it set rock-hard and cold. Once cool, whip it up with a mini-whisk until it is a beautiful white and creamy potion
- You can use it plain or mix in an essential oil or two (up to 50 drops maximum)
- Use a palette knife to transfer the blend to a nice jar

NB. If your blend comes out too hard or too soft for your taste, simply re-melt and add more oil or more cocoa butter. Easy! Feel free to use other plant oils instead of almond, e.g. jojoba, apricot, avocado or coconut.

How to use

Gently press and massage into your face after cleansing. Feel the silky cocoa butter melt into your skin and smell the gorgeous chocolate aroma.

Ingredients

- 50g/1¾ oz organic cocoa butter
- 50-100ml/3½-6¾ tbsp cold-pressed organic almond oil

Optional essential oil blends:

- 25 drops ylang ylang
- 10 drops rose
- 10 drops benzoin essential oil

Or

- 20 drops lavender
- 20 drops geranium
- 10 drops clary sage

Ultimate rosy marshmallow cream delight

Shelf-life: 2 months maximum
Skin types: suitable for oily and sensitive skins

This is a really super-light blend that uses beautiful roses in three different ingredients. It is an ideal moisturiser for those with oilier skins and for those who dislike the heavier-feeling plant butters.

Ingredients

- 50g/1¾ oz organic cocoa butter
- 50-100ml/3½-6¾ tbsp macerated rose oil
- 100ml/6¾ tbsp organic rosewater
- 2 heaped teaspoons gum tragacanth (a plant resin)
- 50 drops pure essential oil of rose (Rose otto)

How to make

- 2 hours in advance, mix the gum tragacanth with rosewater
- Shake frequently for 1-2 hours until it looks thick and milky
- Make the cocoa butter cream using the previous recipe
- Add the rosewater and gum gently to the creamy mixture while stirring
- Keep on whisking until the mixture is light and fluffy, resembling soft marshmallow
- Add the rose essential oil and stir well
- Using a palette knife, put the potion into a nice jar

How to use

Use this super-silky and gorgeously light face moisturiser by massaging gently into the skin until absorbed.

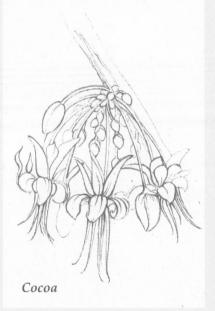

Cocoa

63

Super-gorgeous lavender moisturiser

Shelf-life: 3 months
Skin types: suitable for dry skins

Lavender is renowned for its healing and regenerative properties, and this non-vegan face-cream is similar to old-fashioned 'cold-creams', being super-nourishing yet with a light cool feel on the skin. This moisturiser is ideal as a night cream.

How to make

- Melt wax and heat oil together in a bain-marie
- Remove from heat and whisk until thickened and opaque (but not quite set hard)
- Gently whisk in the lavender flower water until it is a lovely creamy consistency
- Add the essential oil
- Use a palette knife to transfer your moisturiser to a nice glass jar.

Alternative potion: You can change the flower waters and essential oils to make a new potion. For example, try using orange flower water and Neroli (orange blossom) essential oil.

How to use

Gently smooth over the skin after washing or at bedtime to allow this rich cream to do its work.

Ingredients

- 80ml/5½ tbsp macerated lavender oil
- 50ml/3½ tbsp organic lavender flower water
- 20g/¾ oz local beeswax
- 50 drops organic lavender essential oil

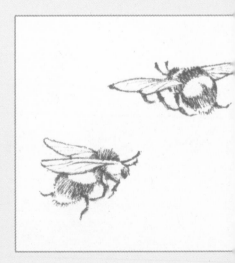

Ultra-silky face oil

Shelf-life: 12 months
Skin types: suitable for all

Ingredients

- 50ml/3½ tbsp almond oil
- 25ml/5 tsp jojoba oil
- 25ml/5 tsp apricot oil
- 20 drops pure rose essential oil
- 10 drops geranium essential oil
- 5 drops clove essential oil

Face-oils are a fabulous way to nourish the skin; they absorb easily and quickly, carrying nutrients and wonderful healing essential oils down to where they're needed. This particular oil has a sexy spicy rose scent.

How to make

- Blend the plant oils in a measuring jug
- Measure in the essential oils
- Stir thoroughly to blend
- Pour into a nice glass bottle

How to use

Warm a small amount of facial oil in your hands, then use light stroking motions to gently massage the oil into the skin. Tissue off the excess after half an hour by gently pressing a clean tissue to the face.

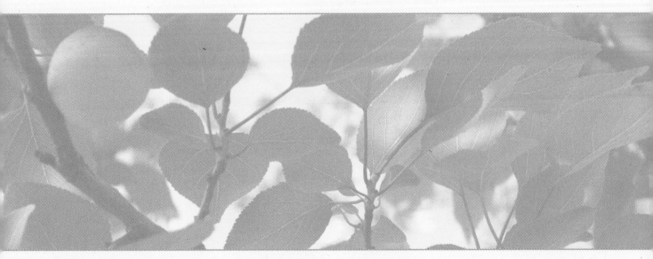

Kiss my vanilla face

Shelf-life: 7 months
Skin type: suitable for all

This face-oil is so yummy you will want to eat it! And while technically being edible, please use it on the skin and make yourself smell as tasty as dessert while the nourishing plant fats get to work.

How to make

- Measure out the coconut oil in a jug
- Chop up the vanilla pod and add to the oil
- Pour blend into a jar and store the jar in a warm place
- Shake the oil every day for 1 week
- Grate the cocoa butter and add that to the blend
- Leave in a warm place for another week, making sure that the cocoa gratings have melted
- Strain the mixture through a funnel lined with a coffee-filter into a jug, and pour into a glass bottle

NB. If the oil starts to turn solid, either store it in a slightly warmer environment or run warm water over the jar to melt the contents.

How to use

Massage a small amount into damp skin to smell like an edible princess.

Ingredients

- 200ml/6¾ fl oz raw coconut oil/fat
- 1 whole vanilla pod
- 50g/1¾ oz raw cocoa butter

Lip treats

Lips are for kissing and communicating verbally with the world. They are made of much thinner skin than the rest of the face, and are prone to drying out, cracking and soreness. Rich and soothing lip-balms create a nourishing barrier from the outside world to keep lips plump and kissable.

Honey, I licked the lips (not vegan)

Shelf-life: 12 months
Skin types: suitable for all

This non-vegan lip-balm contains tasty, lip-softening honey along with beeswax to protect from cracking and drying out.

How to make

- Chop up the beeswax roughly
- Melt together honey, wax and oil in a bain-marie
- Remove carefully from heat
- Pour the molten lip-balm into small pots
- While molten, stir in essential oils using a cocktail stick
- Leave the lids off while cooling

How to use

Apply to the lips as often as needed and try not to keep licking this sweet-tasting balm off!

Ingredients

- 20g/¾ oz natural (preferably local or organic) beeswax
- 25ml/5 tsp organic cold-pressed sunflower oil
- 10ml/2 tsp cold-pressed wild/organic honey

Optional essential oils:
(drops per pot of balm)

- 2 drops sweet orange or
- 2 drops peppermint or
- 2 drops lime

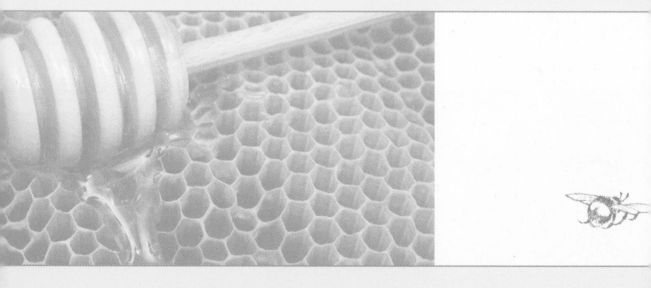

Kissabiliti

Shelf-life: 6 months
Skin types: suitable for all

Ingredients

- 8g/¼ oz mango butter
- 8g/¼ oz wild shea butter
- 2g/¹⁄₁₆ oz organic cocoa butter

Optional:
Add some tasty essential oils, e.g. 1 drop of cinnamon with 1 drop of orange is yummy.

This luxurious lip-balm combines all the best plant butters, for kissing without cruelty.

How to make

- Roughly chop the three butters
- Melt together in a bain-marie
- Stir gently to blend once molten
- Simply pour into little tins/jars and leave to cool
- If adding essential oils, add directly to molten balm in the tin and stir with a cocktail stick

How to use

Apply to the lips as often as needed.

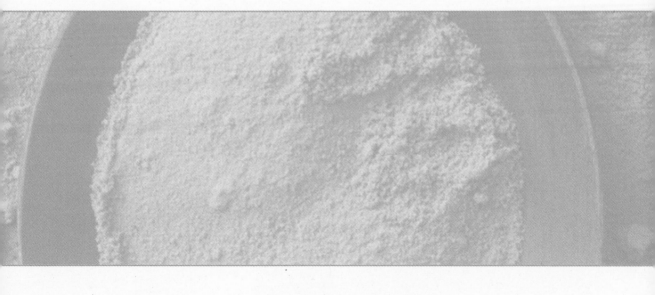

Shea luxury lips

Shelf-life: 12 months
Skin types: suitable for all

This is a very simple balm which uses only one or two ingredients. It is the one I use most often. Shea butter is fabulous for keeping lips nourished and glossy.

How to make

- Roughly chop the shea butter, and melt in the bain-marie
- Once molten, pour into lip-balm pots
- Add the essential oil directly to the molten pot of balm
- Stir to blend with a cocktail stick
- Leave to cool

How to use

Apply to the lips whenever needed. As a former lip-balm junkie, I find that this balm is so rich that I only need to apply it every now and then.

Ingredients

- 10g/⅜ oz fair-trade shea butter

Optional:

- 2 drops (per pot) essential oil of geranium

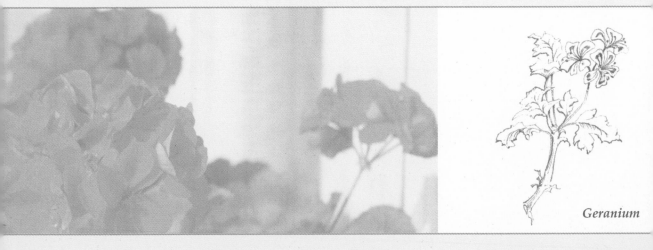

Geranium

In the pink, tinted gloss

Shelf-life: 2 months
Skin types: suitable for all

Ingredients

- 100ml/6¾ tbsp plant glycerine
- 30g/1 oz grated raw beetroot

Tinted lip-gloss is really easy to make, and utilises some of natures best edible dye plants in a base of plant glycerine. It is possible to get really creative and mix up loads of different colours – just experiment!

How to make

- Grate the beetroot and place in a jar
- Pour over the glycerine and shake it up thoroughly
- Leave for a few days to infuse, and shake intermittently as the colour develops
- Once the mixture is a delightful pink colour, strain through a funnel lined with a coffee filter paper
- Decant into a suitable receptacle

How to use

Apply to lips as often as needed for a pretty pink pout.

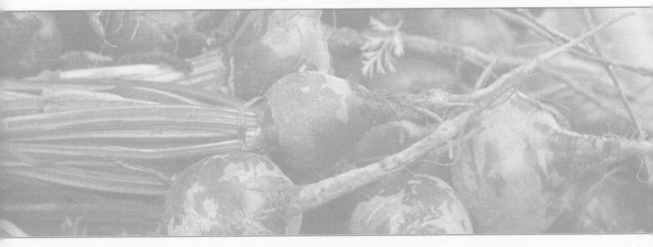

Berry sexy, tinted gloss

Shelf-life: 2 months
Skin types: suitable for all

Another gorgeous colour to try. Just try not to eat the blackberries first – I know it's tempting!

How to make

- Squash the berries and add to a glass jar
- Pour over the glycerine and shake it up thoroughly
- Leave for a few days to infuse, and shake intermittently as the colour develops
- Once the mixture is a delightful purplish colour, strain through a funnel lined with a coffee filter paper
- Decant into a suitable receptacle

How to use

Apply to lips as often as needed for a sultry purple pout. Experiment!

These lip tints are so easy and cheap to make that you can afford to mess around with loads of different combinations of colours. For example, mix beetroot with berries in different amounts to create a whole range of different reds and purples.

There are also other plants that yield colour:

- Lavender will go reddish purple
- Marigolds and carrots create pale orange

Just stay away from anything green (unless you like that look!).

Ingredients

- 100ml/6¾ tbsp plant glycerine
- 30g/1 oz squashed blackberries (or elderberries)

The mouth

Keeping the mouth healthy is very important; it's the start of the digestive tract, and contains the teeth, which are constantly bombarded with all manner of foodstuffs (some natural, some not so). Modern toothpastes contain all kinds of chemicals – and even forms of sugar! The recipes in this section contain tooth-friendly healing ingredients to keep teeth, gums and mouth healthy and sweet.

Clay sparkle

Shelf-life: 2 months (keep very dry!)
Skin types: suitable for all

This toothpaste utilises the cleansing properties of green clay and salt. It also contains myrrh, which is a well-known gum healer.

How to make

- Sieve the clay powder into the bowl, and stir in the salt
- Drizzle in the glycerine, and stir continuously until it is a thick gloopy paste
- Make sure it is nice and smooth – whisk if necessary
- Add the essential oils and blend well
- Put your toothpaste into a jar

How to use

Dip a dry toothbrush into the paste, and brush teeth in the usual way. Rinse well afterwards.

Ingredients

- 28g/1 oz green clay
- 4 teaspoons fine sea salt
- 30-50ml/2-3½ tbsp plant glycerine
- 20 drops peppermint essential oil
- 5 drops myrrh essential oil

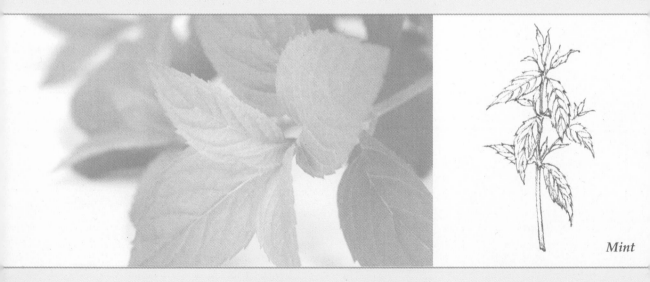

Mint

Shiny smile polish powder

Shelf-life: 6 months (keep water out of the blend!)
Skin types: suitable for all

Ingredients

- 25g/1 oz green clay
- 10g/⅜ oz fine sea salt
- 10g/⅜ oz orris-root powder
- 20g/¾ oz dried mint
- 5g/⁵⁄₃₂ oz clove powder

This is a dry powder to polish teeth for those who don't like the stickiness of glycerine. It also contains breath-freshening herbs like mint and cloves.

How to make

- Grind the dried mint into powder using the coffee grinder
- Add all the ingredients to a bowl and stir thoroughly to blend
- Add more mint and clove if desired
- Spoon the scented powder into the shaker

How to use

Moisten toothbrush and shake enough powder to cover the bristles. Brush teeth in the usual way and rinse well.

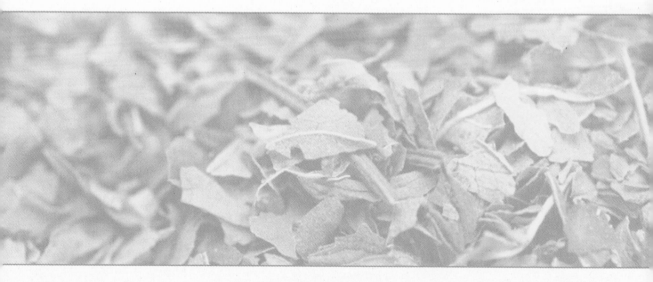

75

Witchy magic mouth

Shelf-life: 3 months
Skin types: suitable for all

This mouthwash uses distilled witch-hazel as a base rather than alcohol, which is very drying to the mucous membranes.

How to make

- In a jug, mix the witch-hazel and peppermint water
- Add the essential oils
- Stir well to blend, then bottle

How to use

Add a splash (approximately 20ml/4 tsp) to a cup of cold water and use as a rinse after brushing teeth.

Ingredients

- 150ml/5 fl oz distilled witch-hazel
- 50ml/3½ tbsp peppermint water
- 30 drops of peppermint essential oil
- 20 drops lemon essential oil
- 10 drops myrrh essential oil

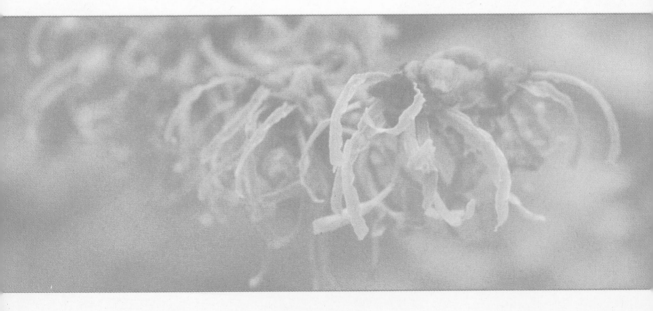

Fruitea mouthwash

Shelf-life: 3 months
Skin types: suitable for all

Ingredients

- 150ml/5 fl oz distilled witch-hazel
- 50ml/3½ tbsp orange peel water
- 20 drops of orange essential oil
- 20 drops lime essential oil
- 20 drops lemon essential oil
- 10 drops tea tree essential oil

This recipe uses the anti-bacterial power of tea tree oil with the zingy tastes of citrus fruits.

How to make

- In a jug, mix the witch-hazel and orange peel
- Add the essential oils
- Stir well to blend, then bottle

How to use

Add a splash (approximately 20ml/4 tsp) to a cup of cold water and use as a rinse after brushing teeth.

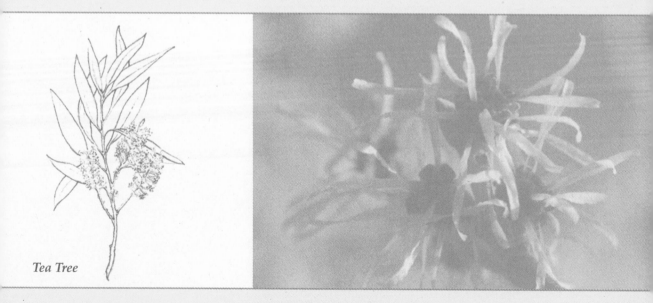

Tea Tree

Masks

FEED YOUR FACE!

A face-mask or face-pack is like a super-food for your face. Used weekly, masks refine, nourish and detoxify the skin, making it sparkling with health. The best thing is that they can be made from normal food items in the fridge or cupboard, and because they are made to be used straight away there is no need to think about packaging or how long they will keep. The recipes in this section are slightly revamped to make them more luxurious, but it is fine to keep it simple and to mix a couple of ingredients, such as yoghurt and oatmeal, to make a face-mask that will work just as well to beautify the skin.

Rose-meal

Shelf-life: make and use fresh
Skin types: suitable for all

Ingredients

- 30g/1 oz fine organic oatmeal
- 30 dried fragrant rose petals
- 50ml/3½ tbsp organic rosewater
- 5 drops rose essential oil (optional)

Variation

Swap rose petals for another herb – lavender is very healing and calming, and chamomile is another skin-soother. Play around and mix up your own version.

This simple and sweetly-scented mask is particularly soothing for sensitive skins and eczema.

How to make

- Grind the rose petals to a powder using the coffee grinder
- Add to a bowl with the oatmeal
- Trickle in the rosewater while stirring until you have a sticky paste
- Now add the rose oil if using, and stir well
- Use immediately as it does not store

How to use

Apply to clean dry face and neck, leave on for 20 minutes, then rinse off thoroughly with warm water and a cloth.

Essential fatty avo

Shelf-life: make and use fresh, do not store
Skin types: suitable for all, especially very dry skin

This is a very rich and nutritious mask, full of vitamin E and suitable for any skin that needs feeding up.

How to make

- Chop the avocado in half and scoop out the flesh into a bowl
- Add all the other ingredients and mash together

How to use

Apply evenly to the clean and dry skin of the face and neck. Lie back and relax for 20 minutes while the ingredients get to work supplying all those skin cells with super-nutrition.

Ingredients

- Half a small ripe avocado
- Small piece of banana
- 2 nettle tea bags
- 1 tsp hemp oil
- 3 tsp apple juice

Variation

For a very quick and simple version, just use an avocado on its own. Mash it up and apply.

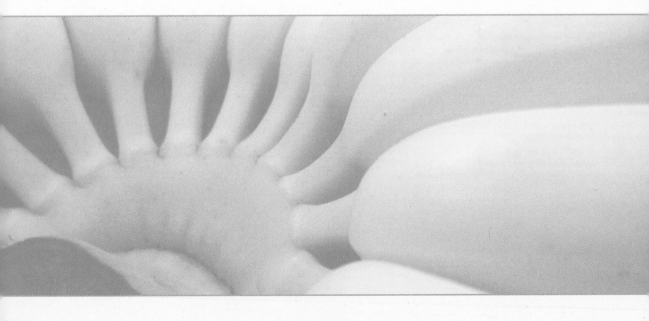

Vera the mermaid

Shelf-life: make and use fresh, do not store
Skin types: suitable for all, especially oily skin

Ingredients

- 50g/1¾ oz kelp powder
- 50ml/3½ tbsp aloe vera gel (either extracted from your own plant or bought from a good supplier)

This quick and easy potion makes a very good all-purpose cooling and soothing non-greasy mask.

How to make

- Put the kelp powder into the bowl
- Slowly add the aloe gel, while stirring
- Mix until it is a thick jelly paste

How to use

Apply the mask evenly to the clean and dry skin of the face and neck. Leave on for 20 minutes, then rinse off thoroughly with warm water.

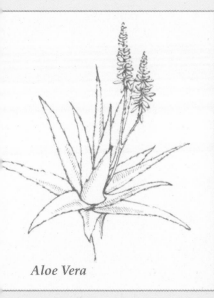

Aloe Vera

81

Glorious mud

Shelf-life: make and use fresh, do not store
Skin types: suitable for all but very dry skin

This is a Moroccan-inspired mask which uses silky rhassoul mud.

How to make

- Grind the rose petals to a powder in the coffee grinder
- Add the petal powder and mud to the mixing bowl
- Trickle in the flower waters slowly while mixing the paste continuously
- Stop adding the liquids when a creamy cake-mix consistency has been achieved
- Add the essential oil, if using

How to use

Apply the mask evenly to the clean and dry skin of the face and neck. Leave on for 20 minutes, then rinse off thoroughly with warm water and a cloth. The skin may feel a little tight afterwards, so moisturise thoroughly with one of the gorgeous plant-butter-based face-creams from this book.

Ingredients

- 50g/1¾ oz rhassoul mud powder
- 50g/1¾ oz dried fragrant rose petals
- 50ml/3½ tbsp orange flower water
- 50ml/3½ tbsp rosewater
- 3 drops Neroli oil (optional)

Variation

Keep it simple by just using the mud mixed with a flower water or herbal tea of your choice

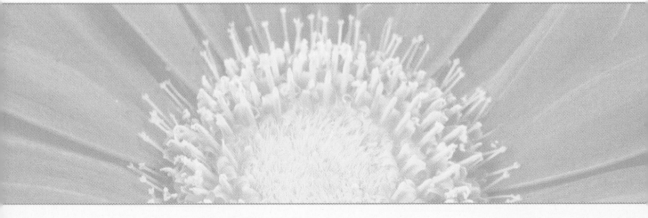

Strawberry smoothie (not vegan)

Shelf-life: make and use fresh, do not store
Skin types: suitable for all

If you can stop yourself from eating it first, it makes a soothing mask – especially if you have sunburn.

Ingredients

- 1 small pot of natural organic yoghurt (cow, goat or sheep)
- 5 organic strawberries

How to make

- Place the ingredients into the bowl
- Mash with a fork until fairly smooth

Variation

Add banana or avocado to the blend.

How to use

Apply the mask evenly to the clean and dry skin of the face and neck. Leave on for 20 minutes, then rinse off thoroughly with warm water.

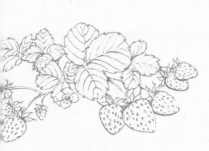

Strawberry

Choc-mud face

Shelf-life: make and use fresh, do not store
Skin types: suitable for all, especially very dry skin

This is a sexy chocolate and vanilla mask full of antioxidants and gorgeous smells, to intoxicate and invigorate even the most tired of complexions.

How to make

- Scrape out the black seeds of the vanilla pod into the coconut milk

- Leave to infuse for half an hour or so

- Blend together the mud and cocoa powders in a bowl

- Slowly add the infused milk while stirring constantly, until it is a creamy but thickish gloop of chocolatey-ness

- No matter how good it smells, please don't eat it!

How to use

Plaster the sexy blend all over your clean and dry face and neck, lie back and inhale the gorgeous smells while the nutritious blend brightens and tones the skin.

Ingredients

- 20g/¾ oz raw organic cocoa powder

- 20g/¾ oz rhassoul mud powder

- 30-50ml/2-3½ tbsp coconut milk

- Half a vanilla pod

the body

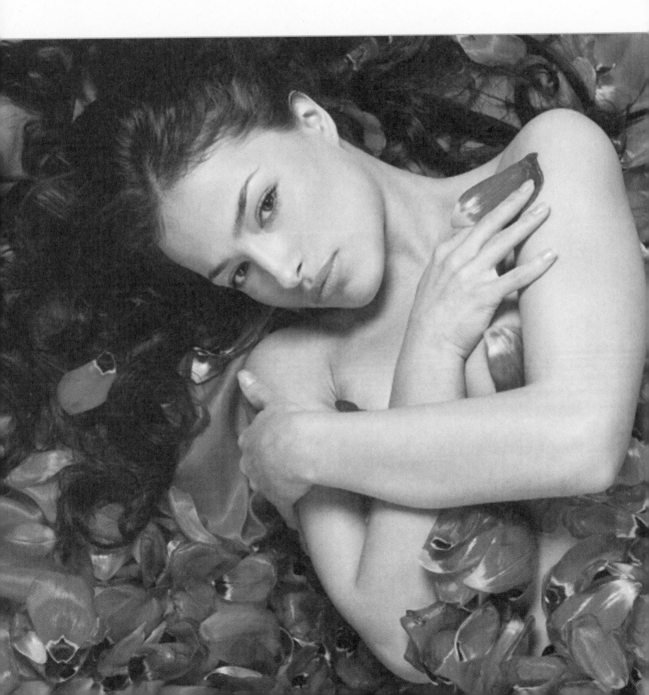

Cleansers and scrubs

It's fascinating to see the vast array of potions that are available for the face, and yet when it comes to the body there is usually much less choice: it boils down to soap or gel to wash with, and some kind of body lotion.

I think that, just as with the face, there should be a veritable parade of superlatively luscious potions to anoint our precious bodies with. Your body deserves it.

Just as with the face, it is better to use the action of gentle plant scrubs than the chemical gels and colourful foaming washes which promise Edenesque raptures of bathroom bliss. Ingredients like oatmeal, ground almonds and sea salt will polish the body, leaving it as silky smooth as a rose petal – even problem areas like dry, cracked elbows and knees.

Mermaid's treat

Shelf-life: 2 months
Skin types: suitable for all, especially very dry skin

Ingredients

- 30g/1 oz kelp powder
- 30g/1 oz fine sea salt
- 50ml/3½ tbsp plant glycerine
- 50-100ml/3½-6¾ tbsp organic sweet almond oil
- 10 drops juniper essential oil
- 10 drops lemon essential oil

This is a detoxifying treatment to be used whenever skin feels sluggish and needs a boost. Containing slippery seaweed and fragrant flower waters, this seasidey treat will make the body feel amazing.

How to make

- Measure the salt and kelp powder into a bowl
- Stir to blend
- Add the glycerine and half the almond oil and mix well
- If the mixture is too stiff, add more oil until a thick gloopy paste is achieved
- Add the essential oils and stir again thoroughly

How to use

Massage the mixture gently over the whole body (avoiding the really sensitive areas) and then rinse off thoroughly.

As an alternative, leave out the salt and turn the scrub into a 'mask' instead. Just apply to the whole body, leave on for at least 20 minutes and rinse.

After eight(ish) chocolate mint scrub

Shelf-life: 3 months
Skin types: suitable for all

This yummy-smelling scrub was invented while presenting this book at a conference; I wanted to show how easy it can be to make a gorgeous product from easily available ingredients (in this case bought *en route* from the tube station to the conference venue). Everyone attending left the building smelling edible.

How to make

- Mix the sugar, cocoa powder and dried peppermint in a bowl
- Gradually add the oil while stirring until a thick paste is achieved
- Store in a jar (Kilner jars look pretty)

How to use

Massage the chocolatey mixture gently all over damp skin; rinse off thoroughly.

Ingredients

- 50g/1¾ oz fair-trade or organic dark brown sugar
- 30g/1 oz organic or raw cocoa powder
- 50g/1¾ oz dried peppermint (or several opened-up peppermint tea bags)
- 100-150ml/3½-5 fl oz virgin coconut oil or butter

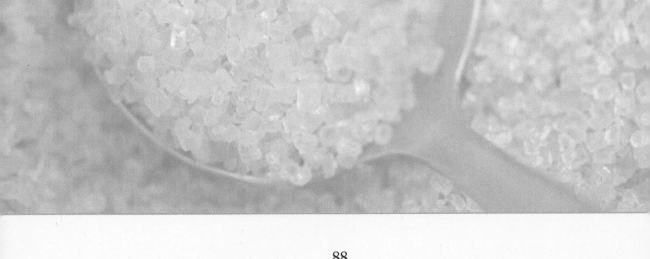

Oaty goodness

Shelf-life: 3 months
Skin types: suitable for all, especially sensitive skin

Ingredients

- 50g/1¾ oz fine oatmeal
- 50g/1¾ oz grated pure vegetable soap
- 50g/1¾ oz dried lavender

Variation

Use other herbs like ground rose petals or ground orange peel, or an exotic blend of your own!

This uses a strange combination of grated soap and oats, among other things. The type of soap to use is a very plain and natural one – try to find a local or online hand-made soap supplier, or buy plain 'Castile' (olive oil) soap.

How to make

- Grate the soap
- Grind the lavender using the coffee grinder
- Mix up all three ingredients in the bowl
- Cut a circle of muslin about the size of a large saucer
- Place a heap of mixture in the middle
- Gather the muslin together like a little sack containing the blend
- Tie it up tightly with the string or raffia
- Store the ready-made bags in a large glass jar

How to use

Use in the shower: soak the little bag under the warm water; it should start to feel squishy and soapy. Use the bag like a bar of soap. The muslin will exfoliate while the oats soothe and the soap cleans. Because the soap is 'diluted' with other ingredients, it is not so drying to the skin.

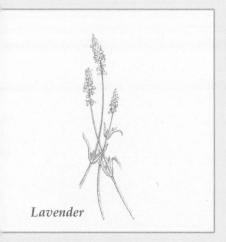

Lavender

Moroccan mud cleanser

Shelf-life: make and use fresh, do not store
Skin types: suitable for all

It may sound strange to wash in mud, but ancient cultures have used various clays and muds to detox and cleanse the body for hundreds of years. This particular mud comes from Morocco, where it has been used to treat many skin conditions as well as in general beauty care.

How to make

- Powder the rose petals in a coffee grinder
- Put all three dry ingredients into a bowl, then stir to blend. Gradually stir in the rose water until you have a silky paste
- Leave to stand for a few minutes for the clay to absorb the water
- Then add more rosewater, if the cleanser is too dry, and stir thoroughly

How to use

Gently massage into damp skin in the shower or bath, then rinse off thoroughly to leave you smelling like a gorgeous Middle-Eastern dessert.

Ingredients

- 50g/1¾ oz rhassoul mud powder
- 50g/1¾ oz dried fragrant rose petals
- 50g/1¾ oz ground organic almonds
- 100-150ml/3½-5 fl oz organic natural rosewater

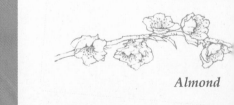

Almond

Turkish delight

Shelf-life: 2 months
Skin types: suitable for all

Smell like a tasty treat with this concoction of honey, rose, vanilla and orange.

Ingredients

- 50g/1¾ oz ground organic almonds
- 30g/1 oz dried organic orange peel
- 50g/1¾ oz dried organic fragrant rose petals
- 1 tsp clove powder
- 1 tsp nutmeg powder
- Half a vanilla pod
- 2 drops essential oil of sweet orange
- 4 drops essential oil of patchouli
- 100ml/6¾ tbsp organic sweet almond oil
- 3 tsp raw honey

Variation

Vegans can replace honey with glycerine, or just leave out the honey and use more almond oil.

How to make

- Grind the dried peel and petals through a coffee grinder
- Place in the mixing bowl with the ground almonds, nutmeg and clove
- Stir everything thoroughly to blend
- Cut open the vanilla pod and scrape the black seeds into the bowl
- Slowly add the almond oil while stirring to mix everything up into a stiff paste
- Add the honey and stir one more time
- Now add your orange and patchouli oils and stir thoroughly to blend

How to use

Massage into damp skin whilst standing in the shower or bath (it can be messy!). Leave on the skin for a while, and then rinse off well. Your skin should feel very silky and moisturised.

Honey & oat cheatin' soap (not vegan)

Shelf-life: 6 months
Skin types: suitable for all

I've never been comfortable with the idea of making soap from scratch, as it uses a really strong chemical called sodium hydroxide, which is a very powerful alkali and can actually burn the skin very badly. (If you've seen the film *Fight Club*, you'll know what I mean!).

This recipe actually makes a new and customised soap from melting down an existing one. In the soap-making world, this process is known as re-batching or hand-milling.

How to make

- Grate your soap very finely
- Place in a bowl with the water and set a side for a couple of hours, stirring now and again. Next place the bowl of soap and water on top of a pan of simmering water
- Add more water if necessary
- Keep the heat as low as possible so that the soap melts very slowly
- Stir gently until it is a stringy gloop (could take up to an hour!)
- Once smooth and molten, add the honey and oatmeal
- Stir in quickly, then straight away pour into moulds
- Leave the soaps to set for 24 hours
- Once set, tip the soap out of the moulds and put on a wire rack to dry out
- Turn over every couple of days, and the soap should be ready to use in 2-4 weeks

How to use

Use with water like everyday soap and remember to rinse well.

Ingredients

- 200g/7 oz plain vegetable soap (i.e. the plain olive oil soap you can find in health food shops)
- 100ml/6¾ tbsp water or herbal tea (cold)
- 30g/1 oz medium organic oatmeal
- 1 tablespoon runny organic honey

Variation

Vegans can still make this soap – for a silky soap, just leave out the honey and add your favourite plant oil instead.

Lotions and butters

As with face moisturisers, commercial body butters and lotions are usually a nasty concoction of cheap petrochemicals and even cheaper plain water. These, along with the preservatives, emulsifiers and synthetic scents, add up to a big bottle of empty promises for your skin and, even worse, some of these chemicals may be harmful. Plus it's a lot of expense for what turns out to be mainly water or mineral oil.

Making gorgeous, fresh and organic body butters which smell divine and make the body good enough to eat is as easy as anything. These pure potions will cost less than their chemical counterparts but will also be full of nourishing natural ingredients that will make your skin super-healthy.

Rosy butter

Shelf-life: 6 months
Skin types: suitable for all, especially dry and mature skin

A simple yet delightful rose-scented body cream.

How to make

- Put the shea butter and infused oil into a food processor

- Blend until smooth and creamy

- Add more infused oil if necessary

- Next add the essential oil and blend once more

- Use a palette knife to transfer your gorgeous potion to a jar

NB. If you don't have a food processor, use a pestle and mortar followed by a whisk instead.

How to use

Massage this rich and creamy potion into damp skin after a bath or shower. Leave to sink in for a few minutes before dressing, so that clothes won't be grease-marked. Use daily for skin as soft as a rose petal.

Ingredients

- 100g/3½ oz shea butter
- 100ml/6¾ tbsp infused rose oil
- 50 drops essential oil of rose

Flower fairy oil

Shelf-life: 6 months
Skin types: suitable for all

Ingredients

* 500ml/1 pint organic cold-pressed plant oil (sunflower or almond are excellent for this)
* Fresh-scented flowers

This is a fun oil to make, as you have to gather the blossoms yourself. Make a real day of it and enjoy all the wonderful fragrances the flowers make; what man-made perfume could beat nature?

How to make

* In spring, gather scented blooms such as hyacinths, jonquil, lilac and jasmine
* At home, strip the plants of any leaves and stems etc. and put just the flowers in a big glass jar
* Use a single flower species or a blend
* Pour on the oil so it covers the blossoms, and place the jar in a warm place
* Shake the jar every day
* Every four or five days strain off the oil and repeat the process with fresh flowers
* After two weeks it should be a gorgeous scented oil
* Continue the process for a further two weeks to make it even stronger if desired. Once scented enough, strain the oil through a sieve
* Strain again through a muslin-lined sieve. Using a funnel, pour the oil into the bottle

NB. Be aware that some people are allergic to natural-scented flowers. It is wise to test the oil on a small area of skin before using all over.

How to use

Massage this light and sweetly fragrant oil into damp skin after a bath or shower, and leave to sink in for a few minutes before dressing so that clothes won't be grease-marked. Use daily for skin as soft as a flower fairy in spring.

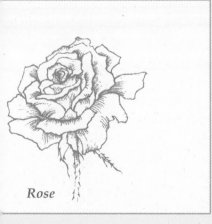

Rose

95

Vanilla whip

Shelf-life: 6 months
Skin types: suitable for all

A gorgeous vanilla butter.

How to make

- Split the vanilla pod lengthways and scrape the seeds into a jam jar
- Add the coconut oil and the scraped-out pod as well
- Leave to infuse for a week in a warm place (an airing cupboard, for example)
- Chop the cocoa butter and start to melt in a bain-marie
- Meanwhile strain off the vanilla oil through a sieve and add to the melting cocoa butter
- Once the blend is totally molten, remove from heat and whisk while cooling until it is a creamy scented potion
- Use the palette knife to fill up the pretty jar with this gorgeous vanilla whip

How to use

Massage this yummy cream into damp skin after a bath or shower. Leave to sink in for a few minutes before dressing so that clothes won't be grease-marked.

Ingredients

- 1 vanilla pod
- 100g/3½ oz organic cocoa butter
- 130ml/4½ fl oz cold-pressed coconut oil

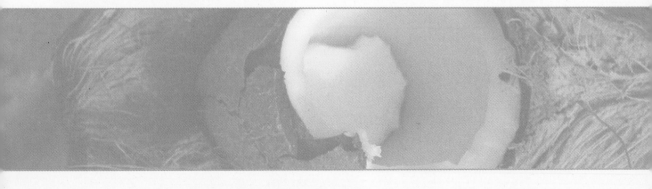

Mango crème

Shelf-life: 6 months
Skin types: suitable for all

This one uses fabulous mango butter, extracted from that large (and annoying) pip in the middle of the fruit. Blended with super-rich avocado oil, it makes a very nourishing cream for dry skin.

Ingredients

- 50g/1¾ oz mango butter
- 50ml/3½ tbsp avocado oil
- 30 drops of essential oil of ylang ylang

How to make

- Chop the mango butter and put it with the avocado oil into a bain-marie
- Once molten, remove the bowl from the bain-marie
- Start whisking the mixture as it cools
- Once it has cooled down and is looking creamy, add the ylang ylang oil
- Continue beating until it has completely cooled to a buttery cream
- Use the palette knife to put the potion in the jar

How to use

Massage this rich and buttery cream into damp skin after a bath or shower. Leave to sink in for a few minutes before dressing so that clothes won't be grease-marked.

Mango

Silky lotion

Shelf-life: 6 months
Skin types: suitable for all

This is more like an oil than a lotion, but it does contain shreds of cocoa butter which melt on the skin when applied.

How to make

- Place the almond oil in a jam jar
- Grate the cocoa butter very finely
- Gently add to the oil while stirring gently with a chopstick
- Slit the vanilla pod, open it up and place in the jam jar with the cinnamon stick
- Put the lid on and place the jar in a bowl of hot water so that the cocoa butter starts melting
- Swirl the jar every few minutes so that it all blends together
- Once all the cocoa butter has melted, place the jar somewhere warm for a week for the vanilla to infuse
- Once oil is beautifully scented, remove the pod and cinnamon stick, and strain the oil into a pretty bottle for storage

How to use

Massage this fragrant oil into damp skin after a bath or shower. Leave to sink in for a few minutes before dressing so that clothes won't be grease-marked.

Ingredients

- 100ml/6¾ tbsp organic sweet almond oil
- 30g/1 oz organic cocoa butter
- 1 vanilla pod
- 1 cinnamon stick

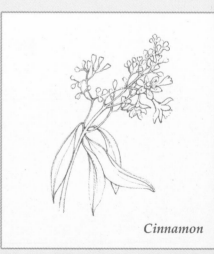

Cinnamon

Shake it up

Shelf-life: 2 months
Skin types: suitable for all

Ingredients

- 50ml/3½ tbsp organic apricot oil
- 50ml/3½ tbsp jojoba oil
- 100ml/6¾ tbsp orange flower water
- 40 drops Neroli essential oil
- 10 drops tangerine essential oil

This lotion separates out into its water and oil constituents and needs shaking (like salad dressing!) to blend each time you use it. Water and oil don't like to mix, and it's almost impossible to make a 100% natural runny lotion as very strong emulsifiers and preservatives are needed. Personally, I would rather have to shake my lotion and know that it was feeding my skin with only the purest of nature's ingredients.

How to make

- Mix the oils and flower water together in a jug
- Add the essential oils
- Use a funnel to pour the blend into a pretty bottle

How to use

Shake it up to blend the oil and water mix, and then apply to clean dry skin with light stroking motions.

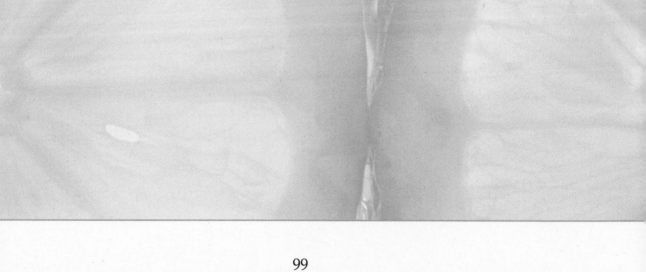

Butter bar

Shelf-life: 6 months
Skin types: suitable for all

This is a solid moisturising bar which can be used for massage or just to make the skin super-silky.

How to make

- Roughly chop the butters
- Melt together in a bain-marie
- Remove from heat
- Pour into a soap mould (or mini cake mould)
- Once the mixture has cooled but is still liquid, you can add any essential oils

How to use

The plant fats in this bar will melt on contact with warm skin, so just stroke the bar over the skin and leave for a few minutes for the oils to sink in.

Ingredients

- 50g/1¾ oz organic cocoa butter
- 25g/1 oz mango butter
- 25g/1 oz fair-trade shea butter
- Essential oils (optional)

Optional essential oil blends:

- Rosemary and lime (5 drops of each per bar)
- Frankincense and rose (5 drops of each per bar)
- Patchouli and orange (5 drops of each per bar)

Sprays and deodorants

So what's the difference between a deodorant and an antiperspirant? Well, technically speaking a deodorant is something that smells nice and covers up the smell of sweat; an antiperspirant is designed to clog the pores to stop the action of the sweat glands. Confusingly, there are also antiperspirant deodorants. Twice the toxicity for the price of one?

In my opinion, antiperspirants have got to rank as one of the leaders in 'anti-health' personal care products. Our bodies sweat for several reasons, and to interfere with this important process is to undermine the innate intelligence of the body and therefore a risky manoeuvre. We should no more stop our bodies sweating than put a cork up our bottoms! Honestly, it's that absurd.

Anyway, what is so wrong with human smell that it needs to be masked? Flowers smell like flowers, humans smell like people. If the interior of the body is sweet and clean, there should be no rank odours arising from the underarms. A water-rich diet of fresh raw foods, plenty of pure water and the wearing of natural fibres (trust me, nylon makes a stink) should be all we need. If you're attracting flies (or worse, suffocating them!), then look to your diet before spraying.

Alcohol, drugs, junk foods and too much processed meat are some of the worst offenders for bad body odour. Not to mention all those lovely anti-health chemicals that are thought to be able to pass through the skin and into the bloodstream – very worrying, considering that the armpit is rich in lymph nodes and is very close to the breast. No surprise then that certain chemicals from cosmetics have been discovered in breast tumours. Of course, there's 'no conclusive evidence' . . .

The best treatment for our underarms is to use sprays made from natural waters and essential oils; this way we can smell sweet without being overpowering and we don't stop the natural action of the sweat glands. These recipes are easy and can be used as underarm or all-over body sprays, and will be gorgeous for hours.

Flower girl

Shelf-life: 2 months
Skin types: suitable for all

This recipe is very flowery and girly.

How to make

- Blend the flower waters in a jug
- Add the essential oils
- Using a funnel, pour the spray mixture into a bottle (preferably one with a spray attachment)

How to use

Spray into underarm area (or all over) as often as needed.

Ingredients

- 100ml/6¾ tbsp rosewater
- 50ml/3½ tbsp lavender water
- 50ml/3½ tbsp geranium water
- 20 drops lavender essential oil
- 20 drops geranium essential oil
- 10 drops lemon essential oil

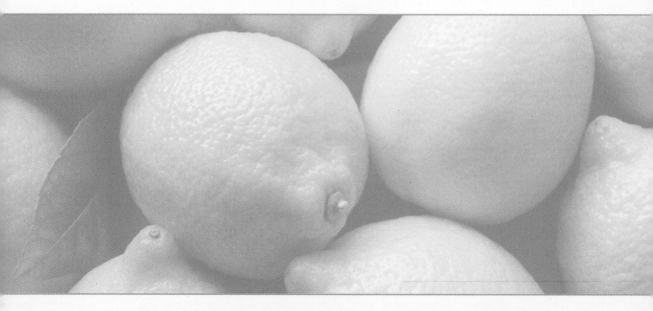

Spicy spray

Shelf-life: 2 months
Skin types: suitable for all

Ingredients

- 100ml/6¾ tbsp frankincense water
- 50ml/3½ tbsp noble fir water
- 50ml/3½ tbsp juniper water
- 20 drops frankincense essential oil
- 10 drops rosemary essential oil
- 10 drops cinnamon essential oil
- 5 drops myrrh essential oil

This is a nice aromatic blend which is suitable for both men and women.

How to make

- Blend the flower waters in a jug
- Add the essential oils
- Using a funnel, pour the spray mixture into a bottle (preferably one with a spray attachment)

How to use

Spray into underarm area (or all over) as often as needed.

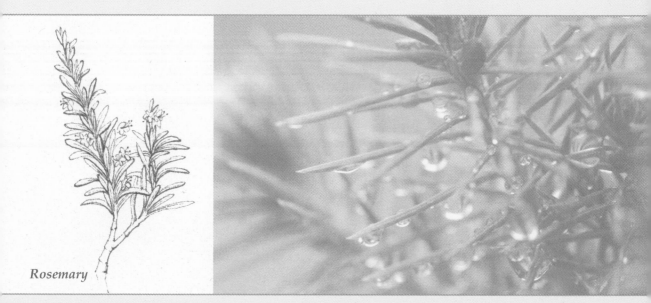

Rosemary

103

Vanilla flower

Shelf-life: 2 months
Skin types: suitable for all

This is a very sweet spray using the evocative fragrance of rose and jasmine with warm sexy vanilla.

How to make

- Blend the flower waters in a jug
- Split the vanilla pod and scrape the seeds into the waters
- Add the essential oils
- Using a funnel, pour the spray mixture into a bottle (preferably one with a spray attachment)

NB. Some people are allergic to benzoin.

How to use

Spray into underarm area (or all over) as often as needed.

Ingredients

- 100ml/6¾ tbsp jasmine water
- 50ml/3½ tbsp witch-hazel water (distilled witch-hazel)
- 50ml/3½ tbsp rosewater
- 20 drops rose essential oil
- 10 drops benzoin essential oil
- 1 vanilla pod

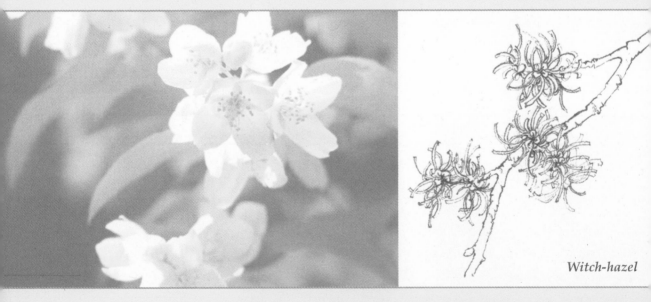

Witch-hazel

Fresh and fruity

Shelf-life: 2 months
Skin types: suitable for all

Ingredients

- 50ml/3½ tbsp orange peel water
- 50ml/3½ tbsp witch-hazel distillate
- 50ml/3½ tbsp lemon peel water
- 50ml/3½ tbsp melissa water
- 20 drops tangerine essential oil
- 20 drops of sweet orange essential oil
- 10 drops lemon essential oil

This is a tangy, citrusy spray.

How to make

- Blend the fruit and flower waters in a jug
- Add the essential oils
- Using a funnel, pour the spray mixture into a bottle (preferably one with a spray attachment)

How to use

Spray into underarm area (or all over) as often as needed.

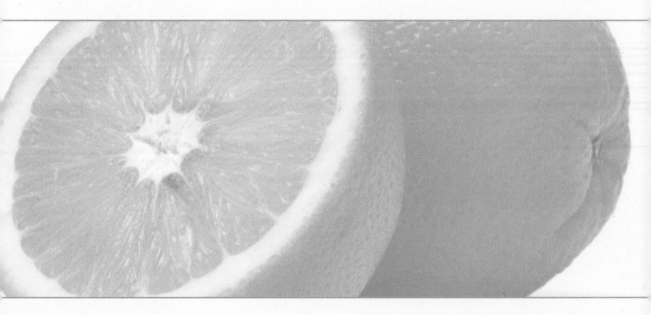

Masks and packs

The body needs to be treated to the deep cleansing of a mask, as well as the face: areas like the back can become greasy and prone to outbreaks of spots; elbows and knees can get dry and cracked. It also makes the skin wonderfully soft and silky, and is a relaxing way to feed the skin with nutrient-rich natural potions.

Seaweed skin-soother

Shelf-life: make and use fresh
Skin types: suitable for all

Ingredients

- 100g/3½ oz Irish moss seaweed
- 300ml/10 fl oz boiling water (or herbal tea, like nettle)
- 2 drops lemon essential oil
- 2 drops rosemary essential oil

This gelatinous mask is great for detoxing the skin and is very cooling and soothing for troubled areas.

How to make

- Break up the Irish moss into small pieces with the fingers
- Place in a measuring jug and pour on the boiling water
- Leave to stand for an hour, stirring every few minutes
- After an hour the seaweed should have gone soft and gelatinous
- Now sieve the mixture into the bowl (force the seaweed through, so that you end up with a greenish jelly-like slime in the bowl)
- Leave to cool until it is tepid, then add the essential oils

How to use

Cover the entire body evenly with the gel and leave on for at least 20 minutes; either lie down on an opened-out bin bag (well, it is rather messy) or stand up. Rinse the seaweed mask off in the shower or bath thoroughly. This blend can be used once a week if desired.

Mud pie and yoghurt (not vegan)

Shelf-life: make and use fresh
Skin types: suitable for all

This is a great blend for calming down inflamed skin and drawing out toxins.

How to make

- Place the rhassoul powder and water into the bowl
- Stir together thoroughly
- Set aside for half an hour for the mud to absorb the water
- Next add the yoghurt to the creamy mud mix and stir again
- Add the essential oils and blend together

How to use

Cover the entire body evenly with the gel and leave on for at least 20 minutes; either lie down on an opened-out bin bag (well, it is rather messy) or stand up. Rinse the mask off in the shower or bath thoroughly. This blend can be used once a week if desired.

Ingredients

- 50g/1¾ oz rhassoul mud powder
- 50ml/3½ tbsp lavender water
- 50g/1¾ oz natural organic yoghurt
- 4 drops of lavender essential oil

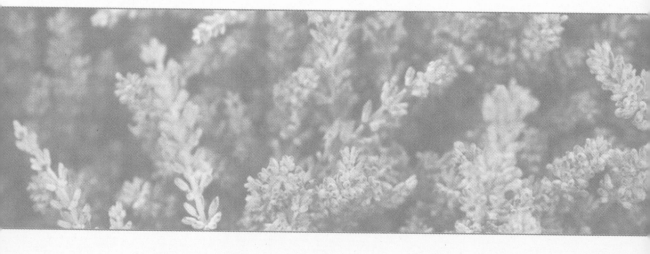

Omega mask

Shelf-life: make and use fresh
Skin types: suitable for all

Ingredients

- 100g/3½ oz organic raw linseeds
- 300ml/10 fl oz hot water or herbal infusion (e.g. nettle tea)
- 100g/3½ oz slippery elm powder
- 5 drops geranium essential oil

This mask uses linseeds, which are rich source of omega fatty acids and are necessary for skin health.

How to make

- Put the linseeds in a jug with the hot infusion
- Leave to cool, stirring occasionally
- Once cooled, strain off into the bowl using the sieve
- Gradually add the slippery elm powder whilst stirring, until it is a thick gel
- Add the essential oil

How to use

Cover the entire body evenly with the gel and leave on for at least 20 minutes; either lie down on an opened-out bin bag or stand up. Rinse the mask off in the shower or bath thoroughly. This blend can be used once a week if desired.

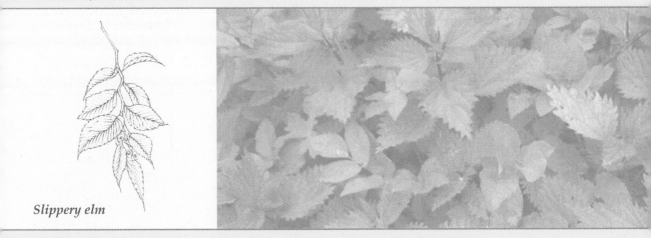

Slippery elm

Deluxe body treatment

Just like with the face, it's a good idea to really pamper the body regularly with a special spa-quality all-over treatment using scrubs, masks and special oils. This intensive body-beautifying normally costs an awful lot; however, as you will be making all the potions yourself with the finest organic and natural ingredients, it will be affordable enough to do once a month at least.

Also it means that you can make the treatment fit your own needs, by making the right combination of potions to suit your skin. Just make sure you have free run of the bathroom for a couple of hours; you don't want to be waiting to shower off a layer of dried-out body-mask!

Remember to prepare everything beforehand so that it is in reach and you don't have to go trekking about the house looking for a flannel etc. Also unplug your phone, switch off MSN and don't answer the door, unless you'd like someone to see you naked apart from the seaweed.

How to make

- Cleanse and exfoliate the body with the scrub, then rinse

- Apply your chosen mask thinly and evenly over the body

- Lie back and relax for 30 minutes; perhaps use a face-mask at the same time

- Rinse the mask off thoroughly in the shower

- Smooth the skin with a tablespoon of cold-pressed oil, to which a drop of favourite essential oil has been added (You may need help with this if you can't reach your back)

- Spritz rosewater all over the body

- Finish by gently massaging in a body butter, paying extra attention to dry or cracked areas

- Finally, look in the mirror and see how gorgeous you are!

Potions from this book needed:
- A body-scrub of your choice
- A body-mask of your choice
- A body-butter of your choice

You will also need:
- Rosewater
- A cold-pressed plant oil (almond, avocado, coconut, jojoba etc.)
- Essential oils of your choice

chapter nine
the hair

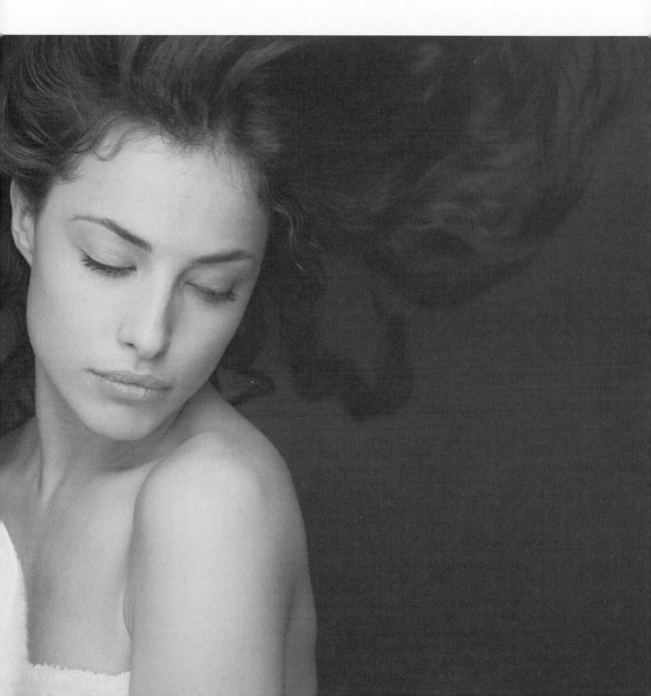

Cleansers

Shampoo is the last thing I would want to put on my hair to wash it. Those bottles of coloured-scented foam contain harsh detergents, some of which are known to cause dermatitis and worse conditions; also, all detergents are synthetic compounds, often manufactured using petrochemicals. Unfortunately, there's just no such thing as a natural detergent; they just don't occur in nature. Clever marketing, however, can lead us to believe otherwise, when labels state things like "sodium lauryl sulphate derived from coconut." This is a cute way to try to cover up the fact that the bottle contains a man-made detergent that has gone through lots of processing, involving such wonderful chemicals as sulphuric acid.

Natural skincare companies can be just as guilty as the big boys of the cosmetic world for making chemical shampoos; it is nigh-on impossible to create a 100% natural shampoo that actually replicates the foaming action of a commercial one, so natural companies either have to shelve their ethics and get on with it, or just simply not make shampoo. Some very well known so-called natural companies shout very loudly about how evil certain detergents are, and yet they make shampoo with similar synthetic detergents that are just as bad.

Some hand-made skincare producers sidestep the issue by making shampoo with liquid soap instead, but again this cannot be considered natural, as soap is also a synthetic product made by a chemical reaction. Soap is also known to be very drying to the skin, and will definitely dry the hair out as well. I have tried it and it left my hair in a horrible condition. The only exception is a soap called African black soap, which is made from shea butter: this is a soft creamy soap which doesn't dry out the skin or hair the way that other soaps do.

So how can we make fabulous hair cleansers that will leave our hair clean, healthy and smelling amazing?

Luckily, there are some awesome ingredients in nature that can do the trick; it's just a case of not trying to replicate a conventional shampoo and being prepared to wash the hair with some odd-looking concoctions! These strange potions will give you fantastic hair, though, so they are well worth making and trying out.

I often get told that I have gorgeous hair, so that gives me the evidence that this stuff really works!

Flowers in the hair

Shelf-life: make and use fresh (the dry blend will keep for 6 months)
Hair types: suitable for all

Ingredients

- 50g/1¾ oz dried soapwort root
- 25g/ 1 oz dried Irish moss seaweed (crushed and crumbled up with your hands)
- 25g/ 1 oz dried herbs suitable for your hair (see list below)

Herbs

- For dark hair use rosemary, sage and black tea (singularly or as a blend)
- For blonde hair use chamomile, dried lemon zest, turmeric and saffron (singularly or as a blend)
- For red hair use marigold, hibiscus and rosehips (singularly or as a blend)

This cleanser uses a pretty pink-flowered plant called soapwort, which actually makes a very mild foam when agitated in water; this is due to the presence of certain glycosides called saponins which the plant contains naturally.

How to make

- Mix up all the dry ingredients in a bowl
- Put the mixture into a jug and pour on 300ml/10 fl oz boiling water
- Leave to cool (stir now and then)
- Strain through a muslin-lined sieve (or a mouli if you have one)
- You may need to be quite forceful and push the liquid through the sieve with a spoon
- You should now have about 200ml/6¾ fl oz of greenish slime

How to use

Fear not the slime, as it washes hair fabulously and leaves it fresh- smelling. Just use it like normal shampoo, but don't expect it to foam up very much. Rinse thoroughly, and allow hair to dry naturally. Feel free to experiment with adding essential oils to scent the potion.

Hair mud

Shelf-life: make and use fresh
Hair types: suitable for all but very dry hair

Strange as it may sound, this Moroccan mud really does clean the hair very well.

How to make

- Add the flower water to the clay in a bowl
- Leave to stand for 5 minutes
- Stir well and add more water if necessary

How to use

Massage the creamy clay through the hair just like shampoo; leave on for a few minutes then rinse out thoroughly.

Ingredients

- 50g/1¾ oz rhassoul mud powder
- 50ml/3½ tbsp flower water or herbal infusion of your choice or from list below

Flower waters/infusions:

- For dark hair – rosemary water or rosemary infusion
- For blonde hair – chamomile water or chamomile infusion
- For red hair – rosewater or rosehip and hibiscus infusion

Variation

Add some essential oils of your choice for a delightful scented cleanser.

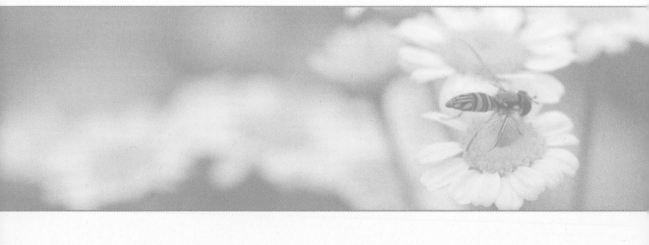

It's the nuts

Shelf-life: make and use fresh
Hair types: suitable for all

This cleanser is made from powdered soapnuts which come from India and contain similar glycosides to soapwort (see p.113.) They don't really lather up, but are brilliant for cleaning the hair and anything else.

Ingredients

- 30g/1 oz soapnut powder
- 50ml/3½ tbsp flower water or herbal infusion (see list below)

Flower waters/infusions:

- For dark hair – rosemary water or rosemary infusion
- For blonde hair – chamomile water or chamomile infusion
- For red hair – rosewater or rosehip and hibiscus infusion

How to make

- Simply mix the water and powder together to make a runny paste
- Adjust amounts if necessary

How to use

Massage through the hair like a shampoo, then rinse off thoroughly.

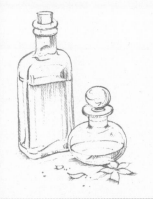
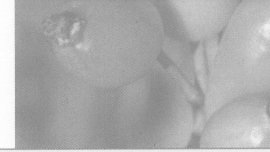

Shea hair soap

Shelf-life: 2 months
Hair types: suitable for all

Normal soaps (even hand-made ones) will dry out the hair, leaving it looking coarse and dull. African black soap (made from shea butter) is the only soap I would recommend for use on the hair; it is very creamy and non-drying.

How to make

- Roughly chop up the soap
- Put in a jug and pour on the herbal infusion
- Leave to stand for an hour, stirring occasionally
- Once cool, stir it until it is thick and creamy
- Transfer to a nice glass bottle

How to use

Massage hair with the cleanser like normal shampoo. Rinse thoroughly.

Ingredients

- 50g/1¾ oz pure African black soap
- 100ml/6¾ tbsp herbal infusion (from list below)
- Essential oils of your choice (optional) to go with the herbal infusion (e.g. chamomile essential oil with chamomile infusion)

Herbal infusions:

- For dark hair – rosemary infusion
- For blonde hair – chamomile infusion
- For red hair – rosehip and hibiscus infusion

Rinses

Hair rinses are the hair equivalent of using a toner on the face after washing; they help to remove the last traces of cleanser and have a gentle astringent effect on the hair, making it sleek and glossy.

The recipes in this section use cider vinegar as the main ingredient. This sounds a little strange, but it has been used in beauty and hair preparations for hundreds of years, and, in case you were wondering, the vinegar smell doesn't linger; in fact, with all the gorgeous essential oils and flower waters you'll be adding, your hair will smell divine.

The rinses also all contain a plant called horsetail. This herb is very rich in a mineral called silica, which is essential for strong and healthy hair.

Raven tresses

Shelf-life: 6 months
Hair types: suitable for all

A herbal rinse for dark hair.

How to make

- Place the herbs and vinegar together in a large jar
- Leave for a week or so to infuse
- Shake/stir daily
- Once the vinegar is scented from the herbs, strain it off through a sieve
- Add the rosemary water and essential oils, then bottle it

How to use

Add a tablespoonful or two to a jug of tepid water and use as a final rinse after washing.

Ingredients

- 400ml/13½ fl oz cider vinegar
- 100ml/6¾ tbsp rosemary water
- 20g/¾ oz dried southernwood
- 20g/¾ oz dried horsetail
- 20g/¾ oz dried sage
- 50 drops rosemary essential oil

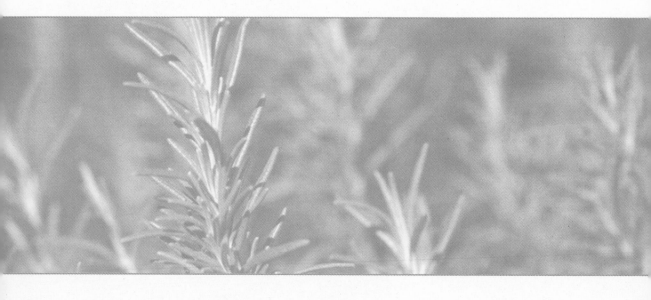

Goldilox

Shelf-life: 6 months
Hair types: suitable for all

Ingredients

- 400ml/13½ fl oz cider vinegar
- 100ml/6¾ tbsp chamomile water
- 20g/¾ oz dried chamomile flowers
- 20g/¾ oz dried horsetail
- 20g/¾ oz dried lemon peel
- 50 drops chamomile essential oil

This rinse is for blonde hair.

How to make

- Place the herbs and vinegar together in a large jar
- Leave for a week or so to infuse
- Shake/stir daily
- Once the vinegar is scented from the herbs, strain it off through a sieve
- Add the chamomile water and essential oil
- Bottle it

How to use

Add a tablespoonful or two to a jug of tepid water and use as a final rinse after washing.

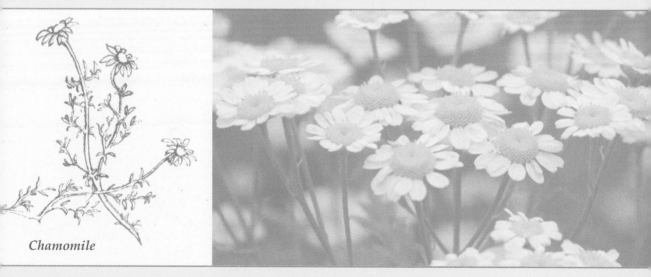

Chamomile

Red rinse

Shelf-life: 6 months
Hair types: suitable for all

This one is obviously for red hair.

How to make

- Place the herbs and vinegar together in a large jar
- Leave for a week or so to infuse
- Shake/stir daily
- Once the vinegar is scented from the herbs, strain it off through a sieve
- Add the chamomile water and essential oil, then bottle it

How to use

Add a tablespoonful or two to a jug of tepid water and use as a final rinse after washing.

Ingredients

- 400ml/13½ fl oz cider vinegar
- 100ml/6¾ tbsp chamomile water
- 20g/¾ oz dried hibiscus flowers
- 20g/¾ oz dried horsetail
- 20g/¾ oz dried marigold petals
- 30 drops sweet orange essential oil

Conditioners

Just as with shampoo, it is almost impossible to create a conditioner that can be applied like a commercial product. This is because 100% natural conditioners rely on ingredients like plant oils and butters but these cannot be used after washing, otherwise the hair will stay greasy; they must be used before washing the hair and are therefore pre-conditioners.

However, because these potions feed and condition the hair so beautifully, it won't be necessary to use a conditioner after washing, particularly if you are using one of the hand-made cleansers too. Within weeks of ditching the chemical shampoos and conditioners you should start to notice a real difference in the health and look of your hair.

Hair guacamole (not vegan)

Shelf-life: make and use fresh
Hair types: suitable for all, especially very dry hair

This rich conditioner uses gorgeous fatty avocados which are packed with vitamin E and protein.

How to make

- Mash all the ingredients together
- Add the essential oil

How to use

Massage into hair, making sure all areas are covered, leave on for 5-10 minutes (or longer if you are patient), then rinse off thoroughly. Next wash the hair with one of the natural hair cleansers and dry naturally.

Ingredients

- 1 organic avocado
- 1 tablespoon organic live yoghurt
- 1 teaspoon hemp oil
- 3 drops lime essential oil

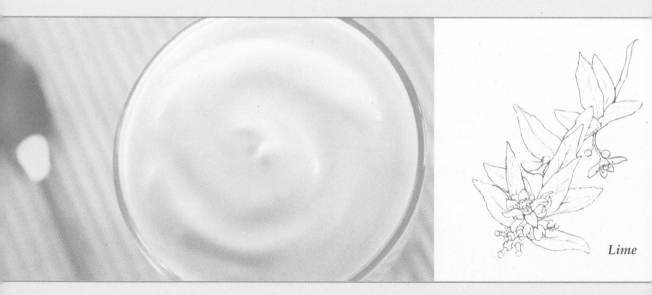

Lime

Tropical hair milk

Shelf-life: 6 months
Hair types: suitable for all

Ingredients

- Half a tin of coconut milk
- 20ml/4 tsp Monoi de Tahiti (Polynesian Monoi oil)
- 5 drops ylang ylang essential oil

Variation

To make it even yummier, you could infuse a vanilla pod in the coconut milk.

This smells lovely and is excellent for the hair: coconut milk contains nourishing properties which will make hair silky and smelling like summer holidays.

How to make

- Stir all the ingredients together in a jug

How to use

Massage into hair, making sure all areas are covered, leave on for 5-10 minutes (or longer if you are patient), then rinse. Next wash the hair with one of the natural hair cleansers and dry naturally.

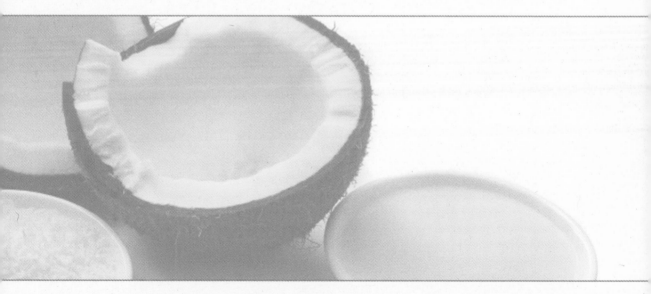

Hot oil treatment

Shelf-life: 6 months
Hair types: suitable for all

This is a really awesome way to treat dry or chemically-treated hair; using the oil hot means that it can really penetrate the hair shaft and repair some of the damage.

How to make

- Place the jojoba, hemp and avocado oils into a bowl
- Place on top of a pan containing just-boiled water
- Let the oil heat up to a temperature that is just bearable on the skin
- Add the essential oil and use immediately while still warm

How to use

Massage into hair, making sure all areas are covered, leave on for 20 minutes with the hair wrapped up in a towel (use an old one that you don't mind getting greasy), then rinse. Next wash the hair with one of the natural hair cleansers and dry naturally. Use regularly, hot oil treatments will give the hair a super shine.

Ingredients

- 15ml/3 tsp jojoba oil
- 15ml/3 tsp avocado oil
- 15ml/3 tsp hemp oil
- 10 drops patchouli oil

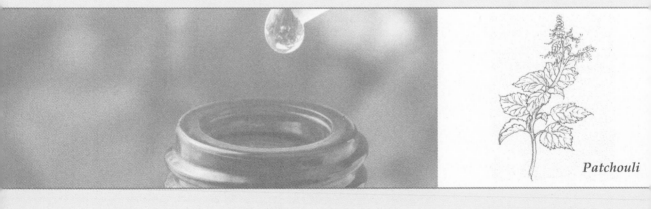

Patchouli

Hair butter

Shelf-life: 6 months
Hair types: suitable for all

Ingredients

- 70g/2½ oz organic cocoa butter
- 30g/1 oz wild-crafted shea butter
- 20ml/4 tsp cold-pressed coconut oil
- 20 drops frankincense essential oil

This is a solid bar to be used on wet hair as a deep conditioning treatment.

How to make

- Melt the cocoa butter, shea butter and coconut oil in a bain-marie
- Remove from heat and pour carefully into a soap mould (or mini cake-tin)
- Once it has cooled but is still liquid, add the frankincense oil and stir
- Leave to set
- Once it is hard, tip it out of the mould and wrap in waxed paper to keep it clean

How to use

This is best used on warm wet hair in the bath or shower, as the warmth will melt the butters so they can get to work. Just smooth the bar over the hair and finger-comb through. Leave on for at least 10 minutes, then wash out with a natural cleanser.

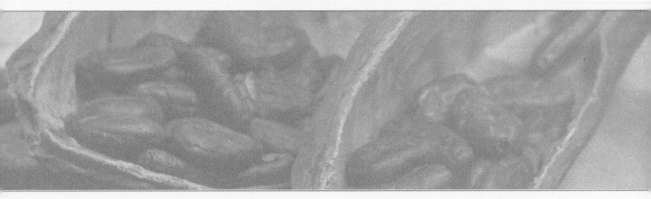

Totally bananas

Shelf-life: make and use immediately
Hair types: suitable for all

Bananas are very soothing for the skin and hair; they are also very nutritious, so eat lots and smear them on your hair too!

How to make

- Mash the banana up with the jojoba oil
- Mix to a cream with the rosewater

How to use

Massage into hair, making sure all areas are covered, leave on for 5-10 minutes (or longer if you are patient), then rinse. Next wash the hair with one of the natural hair cleansers and dry naturally.

Ingredients

- 1 very ripe organic banana
- 30ml/2 tbsp jojoba oil
- 20ml/4 tsp rosewater

chapter ten
the hands and feet

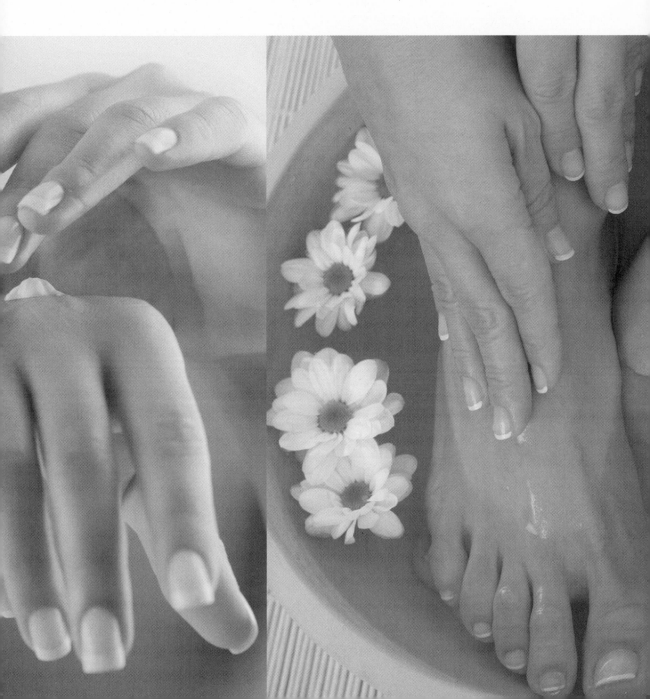

Cleansers and creams

The hands are probably the part of the body that gets exposed to harsh chemicals and the weather the most; no surprise, then, that hands tend to be the part of the body that ages first. They can become very dry and chapped, and can break out in dermatitis from contact with noxious substances. The hands should really be protected by rubber gloves when doing most domestic chores, like doing the washing-up or scouring the bath.

You can keep the hands looking youthful by treating them to some delicious skin food treats, by protecting them from extremes of weather and drying, and from toxic chemicals. Nutritious balms and butters soothe and soften, while gently cleansing scrubs exfoliate and freshen.

The feet, too, are often taken for granted. They carry us about all day, get squished into impractical (and sometimes downright ridiculous) shoes, covered up with nylon and then frowned at and called ugly or smelly! No wonder they are not considered the prettiest body part – look what they have to put up with.

The best treat for feet is to kick off the shoes and socks and let them be naked for a while every day. Even better is to walk in nature barefoot, especially on the beach. This makes the whole body feel amazing, and allows the feet to really breathe and relax. There are several thousand nerve endings on the bottom of the foot, so any special attention you give them will soothe your body, mind and spirit. Plus you'll have the cutest and sweetest-smelling feet around!

Salt of the Earth

Shelf-life: 6 months
Skin types: suitable for all

Ingredients

- 100g/3½ oz fine sea salt
- 100ml/6¾ tbsp (approx) organic cold-pressed sunflower oil
- 30 drops lemon essential oil
- 30 drops lavender essential oil
- 30 drops geranium essential oil

This is an antiseptic cleanser for when hands have been doing lots of dirty work like gardening. A salt scrub is one of the best ways to remove caked-on dirt from hands; not only does it clean effectively, but the salt will also disinfect any wounds sustained. The lemon is anti-bacterial, the lavender is healing and anti-bacterial, while the geranium is soothing to the skin.

How to make

- Add the salt to a bowl
- Trickle in enough oil to make a thick paste
- Next add your essential oils and stir well to blend
- Put the mixture in a glass jar

How to use

Moisten hands and massage about a teaspoonful of the scrub gently into the skin, making sure it gets into all the rough bits. Then simply rinse off. There will be some oil left behind on the skin so you shouldn't need much moisturiser, if any.

Glee – to rub your hands with

Shelf-life: 6 months
Skin types: suitable for all, especially for very dry cracked skin

After using the scrub, use a lovely soothing cream to soften the hands. Rich plant butters are fabulous for using on chapped hands as they are very nourishing and take a while to absorb. You can use plant fats like shea butter or cocoa butter as they are, or make a luxury blend like this one.

How to make

- Roughly chop the plant butters
- Melt together with the oils in a bain-marie
- When fully liquid, remove from heat and let cool (but not solidify)
- Whisk the blend until a lovely fluffy cream
- Add your essential oil blend and mix in thoroughly
- If you wish your cream to be more solid or thinner, then just adjust the amount of sunflower and jojoba oils used
- Now rub your hands with glee!

How to use

Massage a small amount of this rich cream into the hands after washing.

Ingredients

- 10g/⅜ oz cocoa butter
- 20g/¾ oz shea butter
- 20g/¾ oz mango butter
- Approx 50ml/3½ tbsp organic sunflower oil
- Approx 20ml/4 tsp jojoba oil
- 15 drops lemon essential oil
- 15 drops lavender essential oil
- 15 drops geranium essential oil

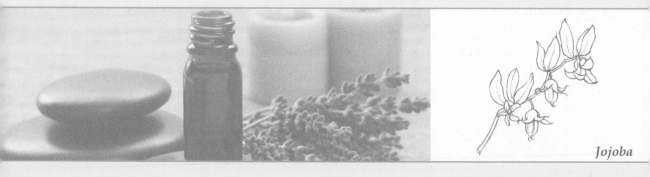

Jojoba

Sleeping beauty soft hands

Shelf-life: 6 months
Skin types: suitable for all

Ingredients

- 50g/1¾ oz shea butter
- 50-100ml/3½-6¾ tbsp avocado oil
- 20 drops rose essential oil
- 20 drops frankincense essential oil

This is a nourishing cream to rub into the hands at night so that it works hard beautifying the hands while you're asleep.

How to make

- Cream up the shea butter in a food processor (or use a pestle and mortar)
- Start to add the oil gradually while carrying on mixing
- When it looks white and soft like semi-molten ice-cream, stop adding the oil
- Give it a final creaming to ensure there are no lumps of shea butter
- At this point you can whip with a mini-whisk to really fluff it up

How to use

Slather on the hands generously before going to bed; ideally cover hands with a pair of white cotton gloves to allow the cream to really penetrate the skin all night.

In the morning your hands will be soft and delicate like a real princess's, and that's just after one night – imagine if you used it weekly.

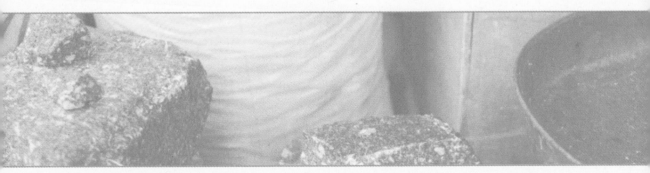

Nine-inch nails

Shelf-life: 3 months
Skin types: suitable for all

While this nail oil won't necessarily make your nails that long, it can make the nails stronger and speed up growth.

How to make

- Put the horsetail and primrose oil into the jar
- Leave in a warm place for a couple of weeks to infuse
- Shake every day
- Strain off the oil and add the essential oil
- Pour into the bottle for storage

How to use

Massage a tiny amount into the nail and cuticle daily for at least six weeks; you should be rewarded with beautiful strong healthy nails.

Ingredients

- 50ml/3½ tbsp evening primrose oil
- 5g/⁵⁄₃₂ oz dried or wild-crafted fresh horsetail
- 5 drops lavender essential oil

Variation

If there is any fungal infection of the nail bed, replace the 5 drops of lavender with 3 drops of tea tree and 2 drops of lavender.

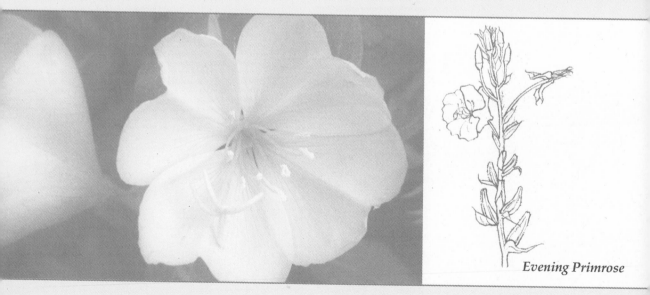

Evening Primrose

Old-fashioned rosy lotion

Shelf-life: 6 months
Skin types: suitable for all, especially oily skin

This is based on a really old recipe for beautiful hands. It is non-greasy and absorbs quickly – perfect for those who aren't keen on the feel of rich buttery creams on their hands.

Ingredients

- 100ml/6¾ tbsp organic rosewater
- 100ml/6¾ tbsp plant glycerine
- 50 drops rose essential oil

How to make

- Simply whisk all the ingredients together in a jug until blended
- Pour into the bottle

Variation

This can also be made with any flower water; try lavender with lavender oil, or melissa water with melissa oil for example.

How to use

Massage a small amount into the hands until absorbed, and delight in having such beautifully scented hands.

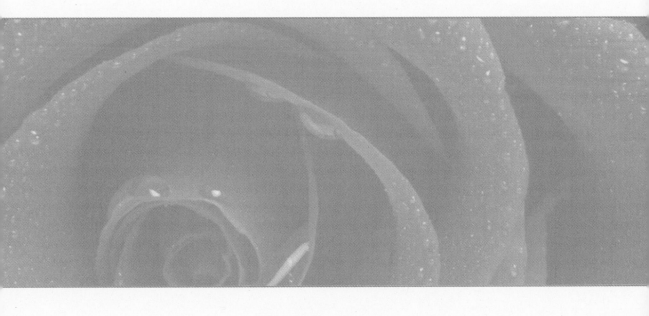

Twinkle toes foot scrub

Shelf-life: 6 months
Skin types: suitable for all

This foot treat makes the skin soft, scented and super-gorgeous.

How to make

- Grind the beans to a powder in the coffee grinder
- Mix with the salt in a bowl
- Add the glycerine and stir
- Then trickle in the oil until you have a thick paste
- Add more oil if necessary
- Now add the essential oils and put the mixture in jar

How to use

Wet the feet and massage the scrub thoroughly into the skin, paying special attention to any cracked or calloused areas. Rinse with warm water.

Ingredients

- 50g/1¾ oz organic adzuki beans
- 20g/¾ oz fine salt
- 40ml/2¾ tbsp organic sunflower oil
- 30ml/2 tbsp plant glycerine
- 20 drops peppermint essential oil
- 10 drops rosemary essential oil
- 10 lavender essential oil

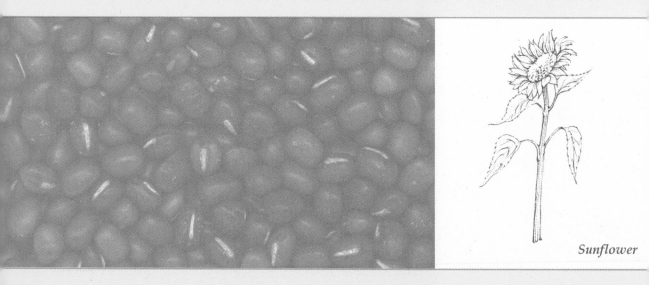

Sunflower

Cool mint lotion

Shelf-life: 2 months
Skin types: suitable for all

Ingredients

- 100ml/6¾ tbsp pure plant glycerine
- 100ml/6¾ tbsp peppermint water
- 50 drops peppermint essential oil

This non-greasy lotion will sink into the skin easily and make feet feel fresh.

How to make

- Blend all the ingredients in the jug
- Whisk until creamy

How to use

Massage into the feet until absorbed.

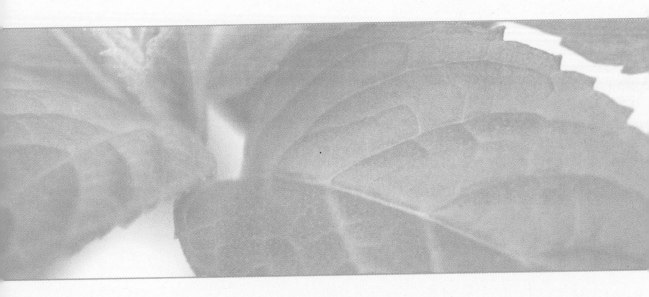

Fruity foot butter

Shelf-life: 6 months
Skin types: suitable for all

This is a rich emollient cream, containing the fats and oils of various fruits, to soften up cracked hard feet.

How to make

- Melt together the fats and oil in a bain-marie
- Remove from heat and whisk until thickened and cool
- Now add the essential oils and whisk again
- Transfer the potion to the glass jar

How to use

Slather on the feet generously, paying attention to very hard and dry areas. This foot butter works really well if you put it on before bed and wear a pair of clean cotton socks to keep the potion in place.

Ingredients

- 35g/1¼ oz mango butter
- 35g/1¼ oz shea butter
- 100ml/6¾ tbsp avocado oil
- 10 drops ginger essential oil
- 20 drops geranium essential oil

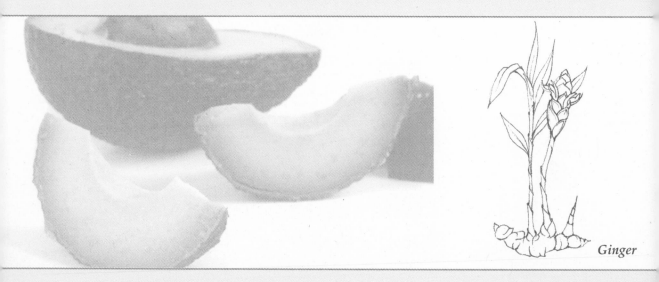

Ginger

Flowery foot spray

Shelf-life: 3 months
Skin types: suitable for all

Ingredients

- 50ml/3½ tbsp witch-hazel water
- 100ml/6¾ tbsp lavender water
- 50ml/3½ tbsp peppermint water
- 20 drops lemon essential oil
- 20 drops geranium essential oil

This is a sweet-smelling mist to spritz onto the feet whenever they need freshening up.

How to make

- Blend all the ingredients together
- Pour into the spray bottle

How to use

Spritz the feet whenever desired.

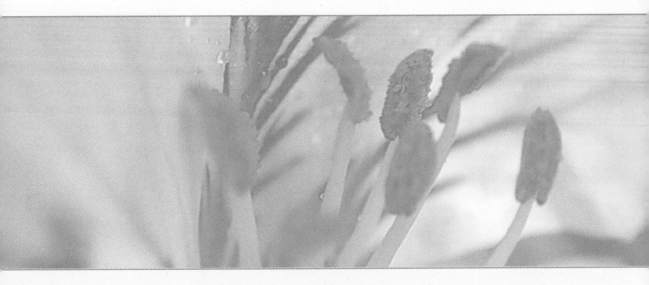

Flowery foot powder

Shelf-life: 6 months
Skin types: suitable for all

This is a healthier alternative to talcum powder, which, shockingly, has been found to often be contaminated with asbestos!

How to make

- Grind the rose petals and lavender into fine powder with the coffee grinder
- Mix well with all the other ingredients
- Keep in a pretty jar or special shaker

How to use

Powder the feet liberally with this sweet mixture daily or whenever you have the urge for fragrant feet.

Ingredients

- 50g/1¾ oz arrowroot powder
- 50g/1¾ oz orris-root powder
- 50g/1¾ oz dried fragrant rose petals
- 50g/1¾ oz dried lavender

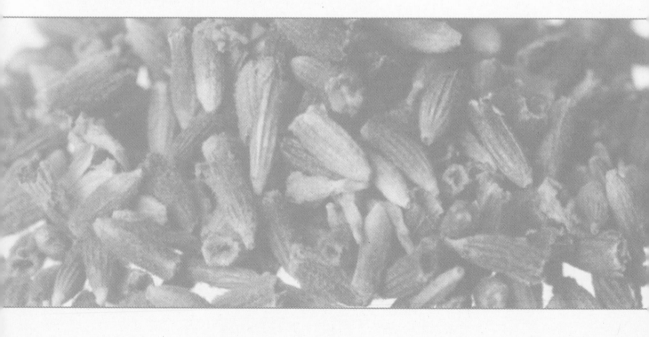

The 'footcial' – like a facial but for the feet

Ingredients

Potions needed:

- Twinkle toes foot-scrub
- Flowery foot spray
- Fruity foot butter

Oils needed:

- Peppermint essential oil
- Avocado oil

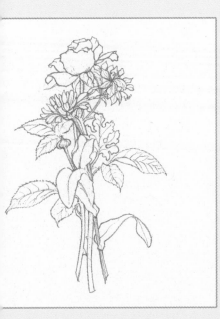

Treat your hard-working feet to this ultimate treatment: unplug your phone and laptop, shut down MSN and give your feet some uninterrupted pampering pleasure. This is ideal to do before bed so that the feet can truly have a good long rest.

It is important to gather all the stuff needed beforehand so you can truly relax and not have to go scurrying off looking for some toe cream or whatnot.

How to make and use

- Fill a big bowl with warm water, add a couple of drops of peppermint essential oil, and soak the feet for about 10 minutes

- Gently rub in some plain avocado oil and place feet back into the warm water (this helps the oil to penetrate the hard thickened areas of skin so they are much easier to scrub off)

- Massage the feet with the Twinkle toes foot-scrub

- Put your freshly scrubbed pink feet back into the water to rinse off any particles

- Using a soft fluffy towel, gently pat your feet dry

- Spritz your feet gently with the flowery foot spray

- Nourish your feet with the fruity foot butter – really slather it on thickly

- Put on a pair of cotton socks so that the cream can get to work softening those hard-working feet. Then either go to bed or put your feet up for at least half an hour

- Afterwards your feet should feel light and silky as if someone has replaced your normal earthy feet with those of a delicate fairy

bathroom bliss

Bathing is a wonderful and relaxing way to wash and care for our skin. We don't need an artillery of brightly coloured, perfumed, foaming liquids to clean our bodies effectively. Toxic bath products are harmful to our skin, and to the environment once they are flushed down the plughole.

Make washing a divine experience by using only 100% hand-made natural and organic potions, and taking enough time out to really enjoy the indulgence. Light some candles, turn off the mobile phone and relax.

Allowing ourselves this time to really care for our bodies is an amazing way to de-stress.

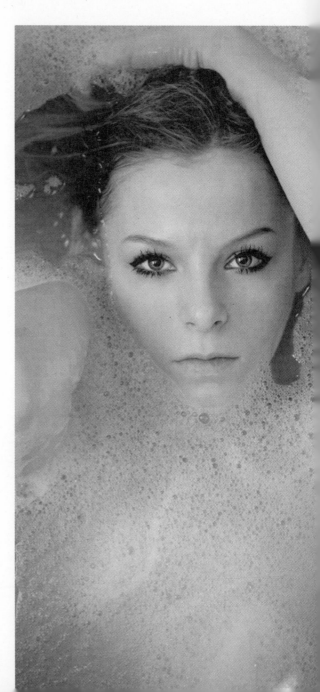

Beautiful bath melts

Shelf-life: 6 months
Skin types: suitable for all

Ingredients

- 100g/3½ oz organic cocoa butter
- 100g/3½ oz dried lavender
- Lavender essential oil (1-2 drops per melt)

Variations

Use 50% cocoa butter and 50% shea butter as your base instead of just plain cocoa butter

Other herb combinations:
Try rose-petals and grated orange zest, or chamomile and marigold for example.

Bath melts are shapes made from cocoa butter and/or other solid plant fats which can be blended with herbs, dried flowers or essential oils. They melt in a warm bath and coat the body in a moisturising layer of plant butter. Silky and divine!

How to make

- Roughly chop the cocoa butter and add to the bain-marie
- Stir it until melted
- Once molten remove from the heat
- Put the dried lavender into some ice-cube trays (funky shapes like hearts are nice!)
- Fill each shape up about halfway, then carefully pour in your melted cocoa butter
- Add any essential oils – 1-2 drops per melt
- Put the tray into the fridge or set aside until solid
- Once set, store the melts in a jar
- I like to decorate mine with a rosebud – I just push it in before they set

How to use

Use one melt per bath; be careful as they can make the bath slippery. They can also be popped inside a muslin bag first; that way you get all the benefits without the bits.

Pretty petals bath salts

Shelf-life: 6 months
Skin types: suitable for all

These are easy and quick to make and look very pretty in the jar and in the bath. They are excellent as gifts to friends and family.

How to make

- Mix the herbs and salt in the bowl
- Use your hands to rub the mix together (this bruises the herbs and so more of the fragrance comes out)
- Put your mix in a nice jar

How to use

Just chuck a good helping of salts to a running warm bath.

Ingredients

- 200g/7 oz coarse sea salt
- 200g/7 oz dried lavender, melissa, marigold petals and rosemary

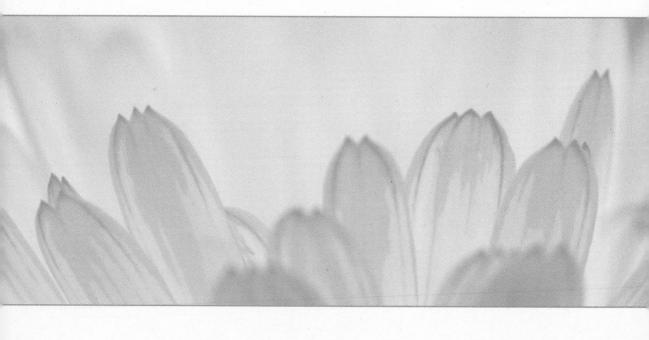

Spicy rose bath powder

Shelf-life: 6 months
Skin types: suitable for all

Ingredients

- 100g/3½ oz fine sea salt
- 100g/3½ oz fragrant rose petals
- 20g/¾ oz clove powder
- 20g/¾ oz cinnamon powder
- 50 drops rose essential oil

This is another bath salt; the only difference is that it is finely powdered.

How to make

- Grind the rose petals to a fine powder in a coffee grinder
- Mix the dry ingredients in the bowl
- Add the essential oil while stirring
- Put the salts in a pretty jar

How to use

Chuck a handful of spicy salts into a warm bath and swish the water about to dissolve the salt.

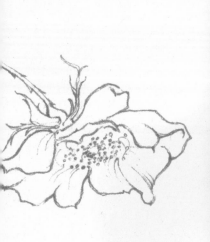

Rose

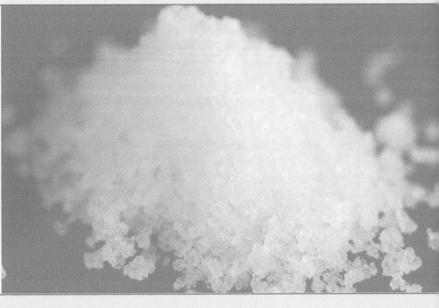

Luxury creamy salts

Shelf-life: 6 months
Skin types: suitable for all

These are the sexiest bath salts ever!

How to make

- Split the vanilla pod lengthways
- Scrape the seeds out into the bowl with the salt
- Finely grate the cocoa butter and mix with the salt and vanilla seeds
- Now add the essential oils and stir really well to blend
- Transfer the mixture to a jar and leave for a few days to infuse before using

How to use

Chuck a handful into a warm bath and swish the water about to dissolve the salt.

Ingredients

- 100g/3½ oz coarse sea salts
- 1 vanilla pod
- 50g/1¾ oz cocoa butter
- 30 drops patchouli essential oil
- 10 drops ylang ylang essential oil

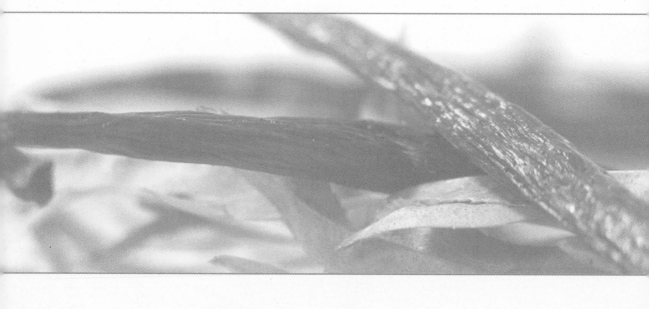

Angel dust

Shelf-life: 6 months
Skin types: suitable for all

Ingredients

- 50g/1¾ oz bicarbonate of soda
- 50g/1¾ oz citric acid
- 30 drops jasmine essential oil

This is a fizzy powder to make bath-time a magical experience.

How to make

- Mix the two powders in the bowl
- Add the jasmine oil while stirring to blend

How to use

Put a tablespoon of fizzy powder in a warm bath.

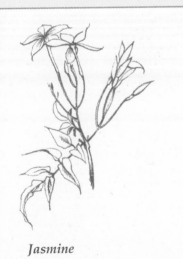

Jasmine

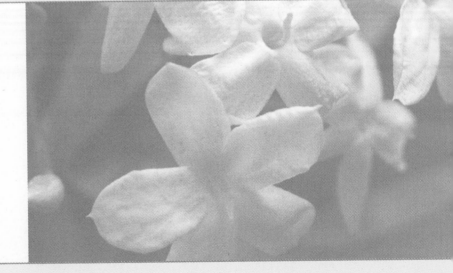

Spicy bath truffles

Shelf-life: 6 months
Skin types: suitable for all

These cute little bath treats are ideal as gifts for friends and family. You could put them into mini muffin cases and decorate the tops with a clove or a curl of orange peel. Just remember to say that they are for the bath!

How to make

- Put all the dry ingredients into a bowl
- Add shea butter lumps and rub into the mix with your fingers (like making pastry)
- Keep on doing this until the mixture sticks together nicely and holds a shape
- Divide the mixture up into truffle-sized lumps and roll up into neat balls
- Put them into the fridge to harden up a bit, then stick them in a jar to store

How to use

Either drop a truffle in the bath and let it melt (you can put it in a muslin bag first so the bits don't stick to your skin) or moisten it and use like a body-scrub.

Ingredients

- 100g/3½ oz fine oatmeal
- 50g/1¾ oz ground almonds
- 50-100g/1¾-3½ oz shea butter roughly chopped
- 1 tsp ground cinnamon
- 1 tsp ground ginger
- 1 tsp ground cloves
- 1 tsp ground nutmeg
- 3 tsp finely grated fresh orange zest

Variations

Roll the balls on some dried spice or rose petals to further decorate them. Put each one into a mini muffin case to present as a gift.

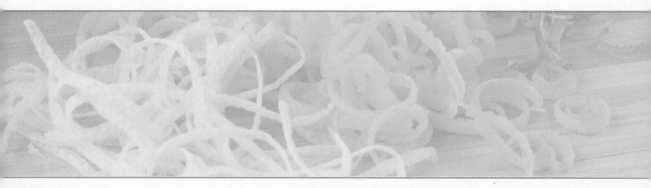

Winter truffles

Shelf-life: 6 months
Skin types: suitable for all

Ingredients

- 100g/3½ oz fine oatmeal
- 50g/1¾ oz ground almonds
- 50-100g/1¾-3½ oz shea butter roughly chopped
- 2 tsp powdered frankincense
- 2 tsp powdered myrrh
- 2 tsp gold (just kidding!!)
- 2 tsp powdered bay leaves

These are quite Christmassy, so are ideal as presents, or for when you need to escape the madness of the festive season.

How to make

- Put all the dry ingredients into a bowl
- Add shea butter lumps and rub into the mix with your fingers (like making pastry)
- Keep on doing this until the mixture sticks together nicely and holds a shape
- Divide the mixture up into truffle-sized lumps and roll up into neat balls
- Put them into the fridge to harden up a bit, then stick them in a jar to store

How to use

Either drop a truffle in the bath and let it melt (you can put it in a muslin bag first so the bits don't stick to your skin) or moisten it and use like a body-scrub.

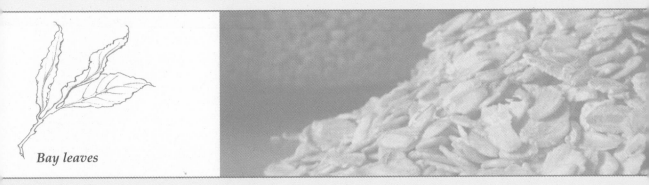

Bay leaves

Flower truffles

Shelf-life: 6 months
Skin types: suitable for all

Cute and spicy flowery truffles.

How to make

- Put all the dry ingredients into a bowl
- Add shea butter lumps and rub into the mix with your fingers (like making pastry)
- Keep on doing this until the mixture sticks together nicely and holds a shape
- Divide the mixture up into truffle-sized lumps and roll up into neat balls
- Put them into the fridge to harden up a bit, then stick them in a jar to store
- Decorate with a rosebud

How to use

Either drop a truffle in the bath and let it melt (you can put it in a muslin bag first so the bits don't stick to your skin) or moisten it and use like a body-scrub.

Ingredients

- 100g/3½ oz fine oatmeal
- 50g/1¾ oz ground almonds
- 50-100g/1¾-3½ oz shea butter (enough to stick everything together)
- 30g/1 oz powdered dried rose petals
- 1 tsp ground cloves
- 1 freshly scraped vanilla pod (or a drop of essence will do)

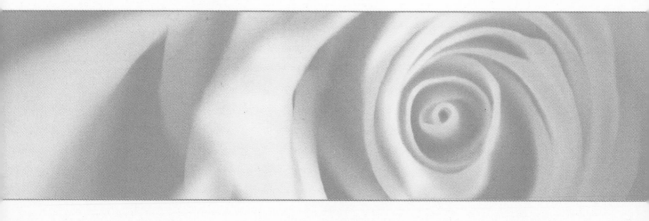

Herbal bath bag

Shelf-life: 3 months, as a dry mix
Skin types: suitable for all, especially those suffering with eczema

Ingredients

- 50g/1¾ oz organic fine oatmeal (or oatmeal and ground almond blend)
- 50g/1¾ oz dried organic lavender

These can be used instead of soap, and are great for sensitive skins.

How to make

- Grind half of the lavender in a coffee grinder, leaving the rest whole
- Mix all ingredients together
- Tie up in a muslin circle with raffia to make a little sack
- You can make several of these up at once and store them in a glass jar

How to use

Add to warm bath and use the oaty bag like soap; once it is wet it will feel a bit slimy – that's the soothing oat-milk coming out. It really does clean effectively, but won't dry skin like soap and is very healing for dry sensitive skin and eczema. Use a bag once only.

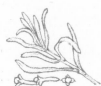

Lavender

Super-silky bath bag

Shelf-life: 3 months
Skin types: suitable for all

A luxurious bath bag using cocoa butter.

How to make

- Grind half of the rose petals in a coffee grinder, leaving the rest whole
- Mix all ingredients together
- Tie up in a muslin circle with raffia to make a little sack
- You can make several of these up at once and store them in a glass jar

How to use

Add to warm bath and use the oaty bag like soap. It really does clean effectively but does not dry skin like soap – the cocoa butter will actually moisturise the skin while bathing.

Ingredients

- 30g/1 oz organic fine oatmeal
- 20g/¾ oz organic ground almonds
- 50g/1¾ oz dried organic rose petals
- 20g/¾ oz grated organic cocoa butter

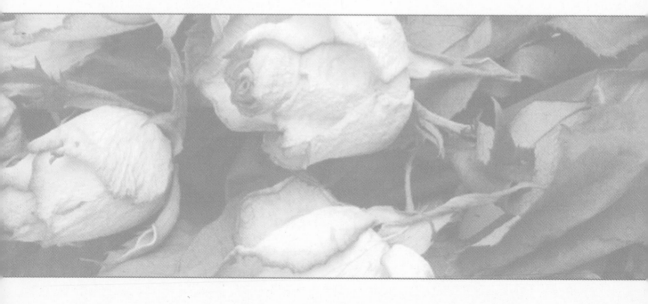

Apothecary bath oil

Shelf-life: 6 months
Skin types: suitable for all

Ingredients

- 50ml/3½ tbsp almond oil
- 25ml/5 tsp coconut oil
- 25ml/5 tsp apricot oil
- 10 drops lavender essential oil
- 10 drops rosemary essential oil
- 5 drops peppermint essential oil
- 5 drops ginger essential oil

Bath oils are a luxurious and skin-softening potion to add to the bath. They are very simple to make, and can also be used as a body oil or massage oil.

How to make

- Add the essential oils to the plant oils in a measuring jug
- Stir thoroughly to blend
- Pour into a nice glass bottle

How to use

Put a teaspoon or two into the bath; swish the water about to disperse the oil. NB: Be careful, as the bath can be slippery afterwards.

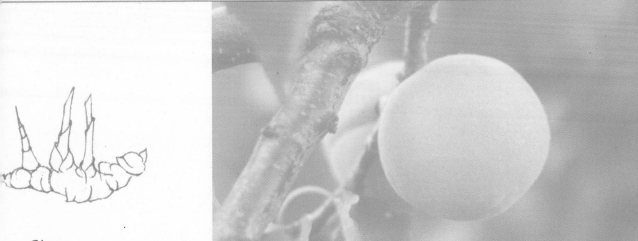

Ginger

Petals from heaven

Shelf-life: 3 months
Skin types: suitable for all

This is a flowery treat for romantic bathing.

How to make

- Combine the flowers together in a mixing bowl
- Store in a pretty jar

How to use

Chuck a handful of these pretty scented flowers into a warm bath and enjoy feeling like Ophelia from that painting by John William Waterhouse.

Ingredients

- 30g/1 oz fragrant dried rose petals
- 30g/1 oz dried jasmine flowers
- 30g/1 oz dried orange blossom
- 30g/1 oz dried lavender buds
- 30g/1 oz dried marigold petals

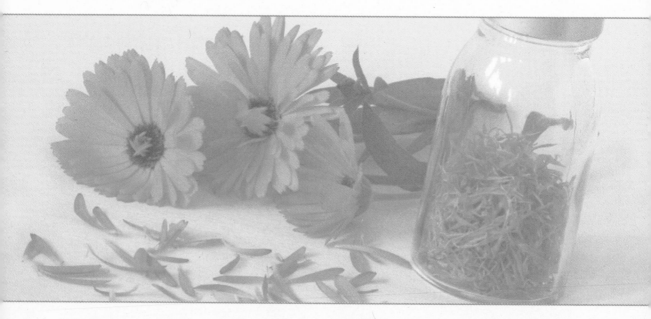

Make bath bombs not war

Shelf-life: 3 months
Skin types: suitable for all

Ingredients

- 60g/2 oz bicarbonate of soda
- 20g/¾ oz citric acid
- Rosewater in a spray bottle (just enough to moisten the bath bomb powders)
- 30g/1 oz fragrant rose petals
- Rosebuds to decorate

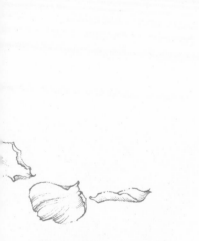

Rose petals

These are fun fizzy treats for bathtime; they contain bicarbonate of soda, which is a good water softener and skin soother. The recipe seems complex, but is quite easy really.

How to make

- Put the bicarb and citric acid in a bowl and mix together
- Powder the rose petals in the coffee grinder and add to the bowl
- Place a few rosebuds to the bottom of a heart-shaped soap mould (or mini cake-tin)
- Then, working quickly, finely spritz the rosewater into your powder and mix it in
- Do not let it get too wet – in fact it shouldn't actually feel wet at all
- Start packing the powder into the mould
- Work in layers, lightly spritzing then tamping down hard before adding another layer
- Carry on in this way until your mould is full
- Make sure it is all packed in and tamped down very well and solid
- Place your bomb in a warm place for an hour or so until it feels crunchy and hard
- Then gently ease the heart-shaped bomb out of the mould
- Place somewhere warm and dry to finish off hardening

How to use

Drop the bomb into the bath for a scented explosion.

Honey and almond bar (not vegan)

Shelf-life: 3 months
Skin types: suitable for all

This is a hybrid bar which combines the action of a scrub with the silkiness of a bath melt; it can be used in the bath or shower.

How to make

- Fill some soap moulds halfway up with ground almonds
- Melt the cocoa butter and honey in a bain-marie
- Pour over the ground almonds in the moulds
- Add the essential oil and leave to set
- Once set, remove from mould and wrap in waxed paper to keep fresh

How to use

In the bath or shower, use the scrubby side to buff the body with, then let the cocoa butter side moisturise.

Ingredients

- 100g/3½ oz organic cocoa butter
- 30g/1 oz ground almonds
- 1 tablespoon raw honey
- 20 drops sweet orange essential oil

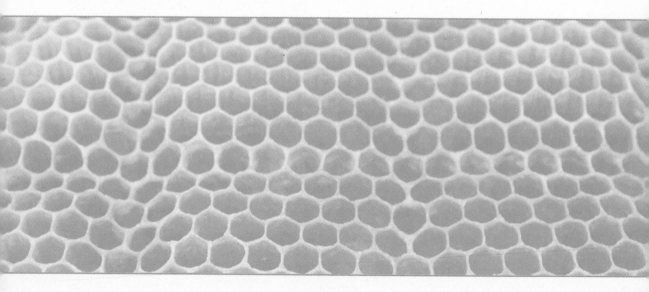

Apricot scrub bar

Shelf-life: 3 months
Skin types: suitable for all

Ingredients

- 100g/3½ oz organic cocoa butter
- 30g/1 oz ground apricot kernels
- 20 drops cinnamon essential oil

A spicy version of the honey and almond hybrid scrub bar.

How to make

- Fill some soap moulds halfway up with the ground apricot kernels
- Melt the cocoa butter in a bain-marie
- Pour melted cocoa butter over the apricot powder in the moulds
- Add the essential oil and leave to set
- Once set, remove from mould and wrap in waxed paper

How to use

In the bath or shower, use the scrubby side to buff the body with then let the cocoa butter side moisturise.

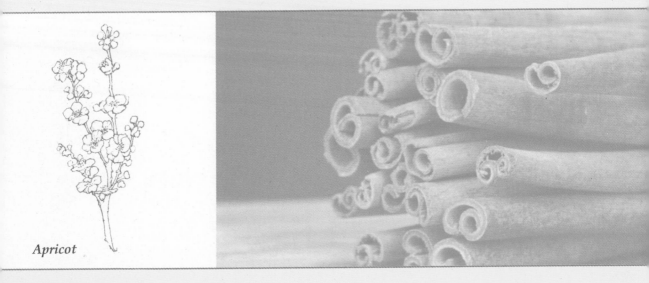

Apricot

chapter twelve
baby and the bump

The sheer amount of lotions and potions available to the new mother is overwhelming. If you believed the shop shelves, then somewhere between tinned purée and plastic nappies the average baby needs several feet of creams, oils, powders and wiping devices. No wonder babies cost so much!

It doesn't have to be this way though. Tiny babies need very little, as they just don't get that dirty (bottom end excluded) – and even when a bit older they don't need much in the way of skincare products. Really they just need something to clean them and then the odd potion for problems like nappy rash.

By making your own organic babycare, you will not only save tons of money, but also will be able to ensure that all products used are baby-friendly and non-toxic. The skin of babies and young children is much more susceptible to being adversely affected by chemicals in cosmetics, so it is wisest not to use them, and to make your own 100% natural versions instead.

You'll notice that there is no cleansing recipe in this section; this is because small babies only really need warm water to get them clean. Even natural skin-scrubs are a bit harsh for their velvet skins, and soap is a bit drying.

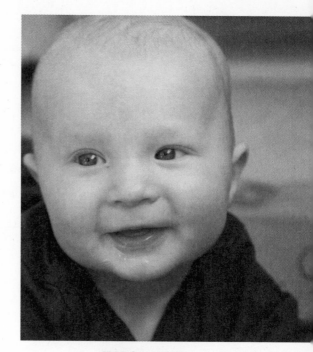

IMPORTANT

- Please remember that babies' delicate skin can even react to the most benign of natural ingredients, so always try out a small bit of hand-made potion first to check for any problems.

- As babies' immune systems aren't fully developed, it's wise to make-up these unpreserved products in small amounts and stick to the shelf-life given.

Wonderful wipes

Shelf-life: 1 month maximum
Skin types: suitable for all

Ingredients

- 50ml/3½ tbsp organic chamomile water
- 50ml/3½ tbsp plant glycerine

These are the holistic version of those chemical wipes that are so ubiquitous in babycare.

How to make

- Mix the two ingredients together well
- Pour into a bottle and really shake up
- Fold up five or so thin organic cloths/flannels and pour on the mixture so each cloth is moist
- Store in a lidded tub
- The liquid will keep for up to two months, but the moist cloths may need to be remade every week

How to use

Wipe grubby hands, faces and bottoms as necessary – no need to rinse.

Belly balm

Shelf-life: 6 months
Skin types: suitable for all

This is designed to make skin supple and to aid stretching of the skin when pregnant.

How to make

- Melt the butter and oils together in a bain-marie
- Pour into a suitable soap mould
- Leave to set
- Once hard, remove from mould and wrap in waxed paper

How to use

Massage over breasts, hips, thighs and tummy at least twice daily.

Ingredients

- 70g/2½ oz organic cocoa butter
- 20ml/4 tsp organic apricot oil
- 10ml/2 tsp organic hemp oil

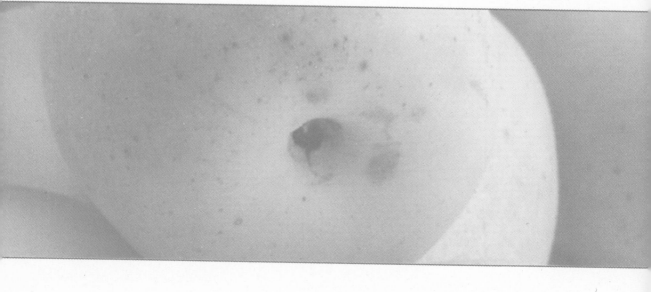

Baby bum butter

Shelf-life: 3 months
Skin types: suitable for all, especially sore, cracked and inflamed skin

Ingredients

- 50g/1¾ oz fair-trade organic shea butter
- 50ml/3½ tbsp jojoba oil
- 2 drops organic chamomile essential oil
- 2 drops organic lavender essential oil

Use on sore areas to prevent or heal nappy rash.

How to make

- Blend the shea butter and jojoba in a food processor until creamy and smooth
- Add the essential oils and blend again
- Transfer to a clean glass jar

How to use

Smooth small amounts into the sore areas of skin after nappy-changing and any time the skin seems very dry or sore.

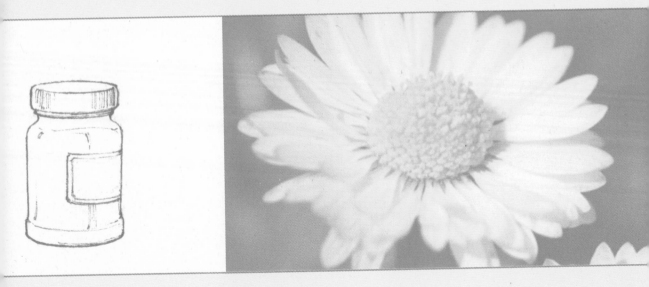

Talcum just ain't welcome

Shelf-life: 3 months
Skin types: not suitable for very dry cracked skin

Real talc is often contaminated with asbestos, and has been known to cause respiratory disorders. If you like to use a baby powder, use this plant-based organic version instead.

How to make

- Mix the arrowroot and orris-root powders together
- Powder the lavender in a coffee grinder, and sieve it so it's ultra-fine
- Blend all powders together
- Store in a powder shaker

How to use

Use the same way as talc.

Ingredients

- 50g/1¾ oz organic arrowroot powder
- 30g/1 oz organic orris-root powder
- 20g/¾ oz powdered lavender flowers

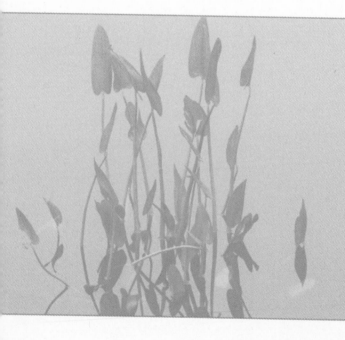

Angel oil

Shelf-life: 3 months
Skin types: suitable for all

Ingredients

- 30ml/2 tbsp organic jojoba oil
- 30ml/2 tbsp organic apricot kernel oil
- 40ml/2¾ tbsp organic macerated calendula oil

Traditional baby oil is made from petroleum products; these mineral oils do not penetrate the skin but form a greasy coating on the surface. Use nourishing plant oils instead for your little angel.

How to make

- Blend all the oils together
- Store in a glass bottle

How to use

Use on sore or dry skin as you would baby oil.

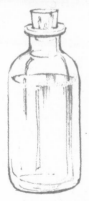

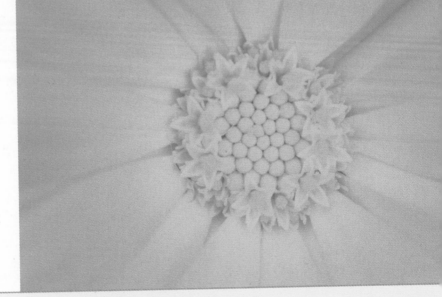

chocolate potions

chocolate

Making beauty potions from chocolate sounds a little crazy. However, there are now many conventional skincare products in the market utilising the rejuvenating and skin-softening properties of cacao. There are even spas dedicated to covering their clients with a variety of exotic chocolatey concoctions.

The only problem is that with 100% natural chocolate potions, it is tempting to try to eat them!

The best chocolate potions are made using only raw cacao, as this has been extracted at very low temperatures and thus retains its nutritional properties.

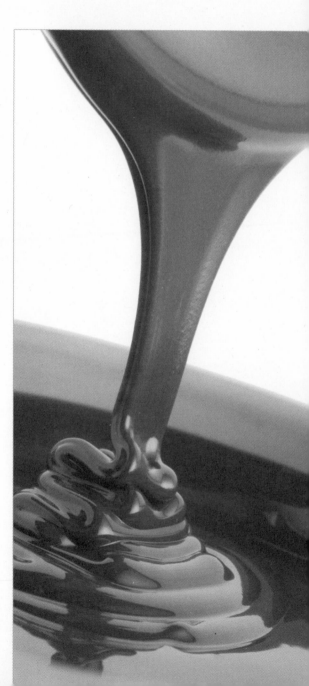

Chocolate body oil

Shelf-life: 6 months
Skin types: suitable for all

Ingredients

- 100ml/6¾ tbsp raw coconut oil
- 30g/1 oz raw cocoa butter
- 20g/¾ oz raw cocoa powder
- 1 vanilla pod (split lengthways)

This gorgeous oil is so tasty that once you've applied it, someone is bound to come along and lick it off!

How to make

- Grate the cocoa butter
- Place in jar along with the coconut oil, vanilla pod and the cocoa powder
- Place the jar in a warm place for two weeks
- Shake several times a day until scented like the best chocolate bar in the world
- Strain the oil through the sieve and pour into the bottle using the funnel
- The vanilla pod will keep producing scent and can stay in the bottle as decoration

How to use

Massage all over the body or dribble a dessertspoonful into the bath.

Chocolate orange body butter bar

Shelf-life: 6 months
Skin types: suitable for all

A solid massage bar which smells good enough to eat.

How to make

- Melt the cocoa butter gently in a bain-marie
- Grind the peel to a powder in the coffee grinder
- Once melted, remove the cocoa butter from heat
- Stir in all the other ingredients
- Pour straight into soap moulds and leave to cool
- Once set, wrap in greaseproof paper

How to use

Smooth over the body; the cocoa butter will melt and be easily absorbed into the skin. You will also smell divine.

Ingredients

- 100g/3½ oz raw cocoa butter
- 20g/¾ oz raw cocoa powder
- 20g/¾ oz dried organic orange peel
- 20 drops sweet orange essential oil

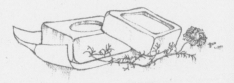

Kiss my chocolate body

Shelf-life: 3 months
Skin types: suitable for all

Ingredients

- 20g/¾ oz grated raw cocoa butter
- 20g/¾ oz raw cacao powder
- 30g/1 oz ground organic hempseeds
- 30g/1 oz ground organic almonds
- 50g/1¾ oz (approx) raw coconut butter

This is a super-sexy raw chocolate body-scrub.

How to make

- Grate the cocoa butter
- Grind the hempseeds and almonds using a coffee grinder
- Mix everything together in a bowl to make a thick paste
- Add more coconut oil if necessary
- Place in a nice fat jar

How to use

Massage into damp skin, then rinse thoroughly.

chapter fourteen
love potions

A little something exotic for when you're feeling romantic!

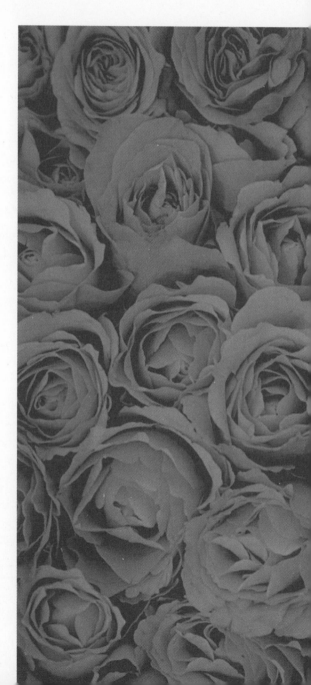

Love spread

Shelf-life: 6 months
Skin types: suitable for all

Ingredients

- 80g/2¾ oz organic cocoa butter
- 20g/¾ oz fair-trade shea butter
- 30ml/2 tbsp Monoi de Tahiti oil
- Rosebuds to decorate (optional)

This cute heart-shaped massage bar uses intoxicating Monoi de Tahiti, which is coconut oil infused with fragrant gardenia petals.

How to make

- Roughly chop the shea and cocoa butters
- Melt gently in a bain-marie
- Add the Monoi de Tahiti oil and warm through so everything is melted
- Pour into a heart-shaped soap mould (or mini cake tin)
- Leave to set
- Once it has started going a little solid, poke some rosebuds in the top so it looks pretty

How to use

Smooth over your body or someone else's!

Fairy dust

Shelf-life: 3 months
Skin types: suitable for all

This is a deliciously scented body powder, which can also be used to sprinkle on bedding etc. to make it smell nice.

How to make

- Grind the flowers to a fine powder using a coffee grinder
- Blend everything together evenly
- Store in a nice jar with a fluffy powder puff or recycle an old talc shaker

How to use

Dust a fine layer over the body and enjoy being as fragrant as summer flowers.

Ingredients

- 50g/1¾ oz arrowroot powder
- 50g/1¾ oz orris-root powder
- 30g/1 oz rose petals
- 30g/1 oz jasmine flowers
- 30g/1 oz lavender flowers

Resources

SUPPLIERS

UK

These are the suppliers that I use. All of them stock some (or lots) of organic, fair-trade and 100% natural ingredients.

www.aromantic.co.uk
- Organic dried herbs and flowers
- Organic essential oils
- Organic and unusual cosmetic supplies (such as natural preservatives, loofah particles, clays)

www.neoils.com
- UK-grown and UK-distilled essential oils
- UK-grown and UK-distilled flower waters – some unusual ones

www.phytobotanica.com
- UK-grown and UK-distilled organic essential oils
- UK-grown and UK-distilled flower waters, some really unusual ones
- Plus lots of interesting essential oil research and scientific information

www.organicherbtrading.com
- Organic herbs and flowers
- Organic flower waters

- Organic plant oils
- Organic macerated oils
- Organic cosmetic ingredients (cocoa butter, clay, sea salt etc.)

They also have an ethical trading policy.

www.sheabuttercottage.co.uk
- Community-traded plant fats (shea butter, cocoa butter, mango butter etc.)
- Unusual plant oils (including Monoi de Tahiti)
- Unusual cosmetic ingredients
- lip-balm pots and soap moulds
- 100% genuine African black soap

www.baldwins.co.uk
- Organic dried herbs and flowers
- Organic essential oils
- Flower waters
- Macerated oils
- Cosmetic supplies (such as glycerine, cocoa butter and gum tragacanth)
- Bottles and jars

www.detoxyourworld.com
- Raw cocoa powder
- Raw cocoa butter
- Raw hempseeds (plus other nuts/seeds)

www.jekkasherbfarm.com
- Medicinal herb plants for growing your own

www.soapbasics.co.uk
- Funky soap moulds for making massage bars etc.

www.inasoapnutshell.com
- Indian soapnuts and soapnut powder

www.colouredbottles.co.uk
- They sell really pretty glass bottles and jars

www.funkyraw.com/shop
- Raw (uncooked) ingredients and super-foods

www.fresh-network.com
- Online raw foods/ingredients shop
- Dietary articles and healthy recipes

USA & Canada

www.camdengrey.com
- Essential oils
- Base oils
- Clays
- Bottles

www.eco-natural.com
- Organic essential oils
- Base oils
- Sea salts
- Reusable & recyclable containers

www.essentialaura.com
- Organic essential oils
- Volcanic clays
- Base oils

- Cocoa and shea butters
- Sea salts

www.mulberrycreek.com
- large selection of certified organic herbs in pots

www.sagewomanherbs.com
- Herbs
- Base oils

www.sunrosearomatics.com
- Organically certified essential oils
- Base oils
- Aromatherapy ingredients

Australia & New Zealand

www.sunspirit.com.au
- 100% pure and natural essential oils
- Base oils

www.gardenapothecary.com.au
- Pure essential oils
- Natural perfumes

www.aromasense.co.nz
- Pure essential oils
- Aromatherapy products

RECOMMENDED READING
Beauty and cosmetics

Cosmetics Unmasked
Dr Stephen and Gina Antczak
Thorsons
ISBN 0007105681

Drop Dead Gorgeous
Kim Erickson
Contemporary Books
ISBN 0658017934

The Fragrant Pharmacy
Valerie Ann Worwood
Bantam Books
ISBN 0553403974

Feeding your Skin
Carla Oates
Vermillion
ISBN 9780091922016

The Ultimate Natural Beauty Book
Josephine Fairley
Universe Publishing
ISBN 0789312115

Herbal Beauty
Kitty Campion
Leopard Books
ISBN 0752900501

The Beauty Myth
Naomi Wolfe
Anchor Books
ISBN 0385423977

Feeding your skin

Shazzie's detox delights
Shazzie
Rawcreation Ltd
www.rawcreation.com

Detox your World
Shazzie
Rawcreation Ltd
ISBN 0954397703
www.detoxyourworld.com

Eating for Beauty
David Wolfe
Maul Bros
www.rawfood.com

Raw: The Uncook Book
Juliano
www.fresh-network.com

The Juicing Bible
Pat Crocker and Susan Eagles
Robert Rose Inc.
ISBN 0778800199

Growing herbs

Herbs: Practical Advice on Choosing and Growing Herbs
Aura Garden Guides
ISBN 1901683095

Plants for a Future: Edible and Useful Plants for a Healthier World
Ken Fern
Permanent Publications
ISBN 1856230112
www.permaculture.co.uk

USEFUL WEBSITES

www.starkhechara.co.uk
My own website – with articles, information, recipes and blog.

www.myspace.com/punkfairystar
My myspace page – just for fun!

www.facebook.com
I'm on Facebook too – search for 'Star Khechara'. I also run a Holistic beauty/potion-makers' group on Facebook.

www.safecosmetics.org
The campaign for safe cosmetics.

www.ctpa.org.uk
The Cosmetics, Toiletries and Perfumery Association. Lots of information on the industry including regulations for manufacturers; check out the board of directors to see the kind of people running the show!

www.ewg.org
The Environmental Working Group. See their 'Skin Deep' campaign with a searchable database to discover which nasties are lurking in your cosmetics.

www.hallgold.com/toxic-chemical-ingredients-directory.htm
Another place to find out about cosmetic chemicals and their health effects.

www.buav.org
The British Union for the Abolition of Vivisection. The place to find out about animal-testing for cosmetic use.

www.pfaf.org
Plants for a Future. They have a HUGE database of plants, detailing their medicinal, edible and cosmetic uses. A must see!

www.soilassociation.org
The home of UK organic agriculture. They have a huge library of research and reports about all aspects of organics, including lots of information about organic standards for cosmetics etc.

www.aromamedical.com
Huge amount of information about the aromatherapy industry, lots of research articles about the scientifically studied effects and uses of essential oils.

www.chrissie-wildwood.com
Chrissie is an aromatherapist, author and deep-ecologist. Her website has lots of information about ethical aromatherapy and herbalism.

www.naturalingredient.org
The place to find out about natural ingredients for cosmetic use.

www.hazard.com/msds
A website with a searchable database for looking up the Material Safety Data Sheets for different chemicals, products and ingredients.

www.wen.org.uk
The Women's Environmental Network. They do a lot of research on the chemicals in cosmetics; they post their reports as PDFs which are free to download from their website.

www.theecologist.org
Website of *The Ecologist* magazine. Check out the 'Behind the Label' series by Pat Thomas.

www.oshun.bc.ca/inci.html
International Nomenclature of Cosmetic Ingredients, which provides explanations of the names of ingredients. So next time you're faced with an incomprehensible ingredients list and you're not sure which is natural or chemical, refer to this list which will provide the common name of the plant ingredients and chemical ones so you know what's what.

THE MAGAZINES I WRITE FOR

The Mother
An unashamedly Earth-Motherin' journal featuring articles on eco-lifestyles and holistic parenting. I'm a regular columnist, writing about babycare potions.
www.themothermagazine.co.uk

Funky Raw
A raw food and holistic lifestyle magazine. I wrote the 'potion pages' for two years.
www.funkyraw.com

Permaculture
The home of permaculture in the UK.
www.permaculture.co.uk

Connect
Free independent magazine about green
living and holistic health.
www.connect-magazine.co.uk

The Source
New glossy magazine about eco-lifestyles
– totally free!
www.thesource-southwest.co.uk

TRAINING

Diploma in Holistic Skincare Production
The School of Natural Health Sciences
(SNHS). I'm writing this course, which
will be the UK's only professional accred-
ited course in holistic 'potion-making'.
The SNHS also runs home-study courses
in Aromatherapy, Nutrition and Herbalism
etc. See **www.naturalhealthcourses.com**
for details.

Beauty without costing the Earth
Classes and workshops with me, taught
at Star Mountain – Plymouth's only
holistic community centre, shop and café.
See **www.starmountain.co.uk** for details
Feel free to contact me directly via email
beauty@starkhechara.co.uk

In beauty **xxx Star**

Index